U0307085

中国器官移植发展报告

（2019）

黄洁夫　主编

清华大学出版社
北京

图书在版编目（CIP）数据

中国器官移植发展报告.2019 / 黄洁夫主编.—北京：清华大学出版社，2020.12
ISBN 978-7-302-57002-8

Ⅰ.①中… Ⅱ.①黄… Ⅲ.①器官移植 – 研究报告 – 中国 –2019 Ⅳ.① R617

中国版本图书馆 CIP 数据核字（2020）第 238001 号

责任编辑：孙　宇
封面设计：吴　晋
责任校对：李建庄
责任印制：丛怀宇

出版发行：清华大学出版社
　　　　　网　　址：http：//www.tup.com.cn，http：//www.wqbook.com
　　　　　地　　址：北京清华大学学研大厦 A 座　　邮　　编：100084
　　　　　社总机：010-62770175　　　　　　　　邮　　购：010-62786544
　　　　　投稿与读者服务：010-62776969，c-service@tup.tsinghua.edu.cn
　　　　　质量反馈：010-62772015，zhiliang@tup.tsinghua.edu.cn
印 装 者：小森印刷（北京）有限公司
经　　销：全国新华书店
开　　本：165mm×235mm　　　印　张：7.5　　字　数：103 千字
版　　次：2020 年 12 月第 1 版　　印　次：2020 年 12 月第 1 次印刷
定　　价：49.00 元

产品编号：091050-01

Report on Organ Transplantation Development in China (2019) Editorial Committee

前　言

　　器官移植是 20 世纪生命医学科学的重大进展，经过了从临床实验到临床应用的发展过程，该项技术逐渐成熟，成为治疗终末期器官功能衰竭的有效医疗手段，拯救了众多的器官功能衰竭患者，促进了我国生命医学科学的发展。由于器官移植需要一个可供移植的器官，无论是尸体捐献器官还是亲属捐献的活体器官，均涉及社会、宗教、伦理、政治、法治等深层次问题，与国家的传统文化和社会经济发展密切相关。

　　器官移植事业要扎根本国的传统文化，立足于社会发展阶段的国情，又要遵循全世界公认的伦理准则。2006 年 3 月 16 日，原国家卫生部印发《人体器官移植技术临床应用管理暂行规定》（卫医发〔2006〕94号），要求将移植医院进行技术准入审核，统一标准和严格管理。同年，全国人体器官移植临床应用管理峰会在广州召开，移植界医务人员凝聚器官移植改革共识，发布了《广州宣言》，全国器官移植医疗机构整顿工作正式拉开帷幕。中国政府高度重视发展人体器官捐献与移植事业，在 2007 年 5 月我国第一部《人体器官移植条例》（以下简称《条例》）由国务院正式颁布实施，标志着我国人体器官捐献与移植工作体系建设逐步完善。同年，原卫生部发布《卫生部办公厅关于境外人员申请人体器官移植有关问题的通知》（卫办医发〔2007〕110 号），明确规定"禁止国外公民来中国器官移植旅游"。2010 年，原国家卫生部与中国红十字会总会共同启动了公民逝世后器官捐献工作试点，本着立足于中国社会发展阶段与文化传统基础，建立了中国红十字会作为第三方机构进行器官捐献动员和见证机制，并依据国际通行准则和中国国情，创新性地提出公民逝世后器官捐献的三类死亡判断标准：I 类（脑死亡后器官捐献）;II 类（心脏死亡后器官捐献）；III 类（心脑双死亡后器官捐献），奠定了中国公民逝世后自愿器官捐献死亡判定的理论基础。2011 年，中国出台了《刑法修正案（八）》，严禁器官买卖的行为，并增设"器官买卖罪"，进一步加强了器官捐献的法治化建设。2011 年，中国人体器官分配与共享计算机系统（COTRS）上线运行，通过计算机系统自主分配，明确遵循区域优先、病情危重优先、组织配型优先、儿童匹配优先、血型相同优先、器官捐献者直系亲属优先、稀有机会优先、等待顺序优先等国际器官获取与分配的原则，有序地组建了器官捐献协调员队伍。

经过三年的不懈努力，试点工作取得了成功，总结出一套较为成熟的工作体系，并建立了中国红十字会的国家器官捐献管理中心。2013 年 2 月 25 日，原国家卫生部与中国红十字会正式在全国范围内开展了公民逝世后自愿器官捐献，所有器官移植医院必须获得卫生行政部门的授权，建立器官获取组织（OPO）和器官捐献办公室。同年 8 月，原国家卫生和计划生育委员会出台了《人体捐献器官获取与分配管理规定（试行）》，明确要求各移植医疗机构，严格使用中国人体器官分配与共享计算机系统实施器官分配，任何机构、组织和个人不得在器官分配系统外擅自分配捐献器官，确保人体捐献器官公开、公正、公平、可溯源地分配，并在移植界发布了"杭州决议"。2013 年 12 月 19 日，中央办公厅、国务院办公厅下发《关于党员干部带头推动殡葬改革的意见》，"鼓励党员、干部去世后捐献器官或遗体"。根据党的十八届四中全会"依法治国"的精神，2014 年 12 月 3 日，国家人体器官捐献与移植委员会正式宣布全面禁止使用死囚器官，这项改革举措得到了全社会的热烈响应和国际移植社会的高度赞誉。"十年磨一剑"，我国经过改革逐步建立了包括器官捐献体系、器官获取与分配体系、器官移植医疗服务体系、器官移植质控体系及器官移植监管体系等五大器官捐献与移植体系，并在全社会大力弘扬器官捐献的大爱精神，公平、透明、阳光的公民自愿器官捐献的大气候正在全社会逐步形成。

　　健康是人类的共同追求，世界卫生与健康事业离不开中国持续不懈的努力，中国卫生与健康事业也需要其他国家的支持。近年来，我国逐步加强与各国的交流合作，全面展示了我国器官移植顶层设计、制度建设、法律法规及工作体系，并通过世界卫生组织全球器官移植监测网向国际社会提供有关数据及分析结果，公开透明展示我国人体器官捐献与移植工作成果。中国的改革得到了国际社会的认可和支持。从 2006 年开始，世界器官移植界就有专家来到中国进行帮助和指导，并与中国专家在国际器官移植权威杂志上共同发表了一系列推进改革的文章，包括 2006 年的"广州宣言"、2013 年的"杭州决议"和 2019 年的"昆明宣言"，他们都见证了中国器官移植改革进程，实事求是又客观公正地认可中国器官移植改革所取得的进步。2016 年 8 月，第 26 届世界器官移植协会年会在中国香港举行，这是首次在中国举行的世界器官移植大会。大会第一次邀请中国专家组团参会，黄洁夫教授在大会开幕式上作了大会主旨演讲，向全世界介绍了中国器官移植改革的十年历程。同年 10 月，中国器官移植发展基金会联合多家中外器官捐献移植机构共同主办，在北京人民大会堂金色大厅召开第一届"中国—国际器官捐献大会"，众多国际器官移植协会专家出席并共同见证了中国器官移植正式走向国际社会。2017 年 2 月，中国受邀出席梵蒂冈教皇科学院"反对世界器官贩卖高峰论坛"，面对复杂的国际形势，我国参会代表实事求是地发出中国声音，讲好中国故事，并获得世界各国移植领袖的高度认可，器官捐献与移植的"中国方案"被世界卫生组织誉为"中国对世界移植的创新和贡献"。正如世界卫生组织移植特别工作委员会主席弗兰克·德尔莫尼教授在梵蒂冈会议上讲到，"你们的骨头也是我们的骨头，你们的进步也是我们的进步"，中国逐步融入了世界器官移植大家庭。世界卫生组织主管移植的官员约瑟·雷蒙·努涅斯教授说，"世界器官移植像一艘大船，中国以前不在船上，也不知道中国驶向何方，但从2015年后，中国已经站在了船的中央"。2018年3月，中国的器官移植改革经验在联合国与梵蒂冈教皇科学院共同举办的"践行伦理行动"会议上发表了会议宣言。会议上发布的"梵蒂冈教皇科学院践行伦理道德会议宣言"中提到："中国模式的基本特征体现在中国政府持续改革的坚定决心，以及在黄洁夫教授领导下移植界专业人士与政府通力合作高效落实器官移植改革措施"。2018年5月，中国参加71届世界卫生大会器官移植边会，我国100多名移植专家出席了会议并在大会上，介绍了中国改革经验。世界卫生组织总干事谭德赛博士称赞并感谢中国为世界移植作出的贡献。同年8月，由中国提议建立的"世界卫生组织器官捐献与移植特别工作委员会"在西班牙马德里召开的第27届世界移植大会期间正式成立，31名专家共同组成的世界卫生组织移植特别工作委员会成员，有两位是中国专家，黄洁夫被聘为世界卫生组织移植顾问，中国开始为世界移植全球治理工作贡献中国智慧。

近年来，我国相继出台和建立了利于器官捐献的法规和机制。例如，2016年，国家交通、航空、铁路等六部门联合建立了器官转运的绿色通道，为拯救生命赢得宝贵时间；2017年5月，《中华人民共和国红十字会法》修订，明确要推动器官捐献工作，探索了慈善机构等开展人道主义救助机制。我国器官捐献和移植的数量和质量也得到快速发展。从2015年至2018年，我国器官捐献数量连续3年增加，增幅在22%~47.5%之间，2015年完成公民逝世后器官捐献2,766例；2016年完成公民逝世后器官捐献4,080例；2017年完成公民逝世后器官捐献5,146例；2018年，公民逝世后器官捐献达6,302例，再加上每年公民中亲属间的活体捐献2,200~2,500例，2018年共实施器官移植手术20,201例，移植手术总量居世界第二位，2019 年始，国家卫生健康委员会明确，我国器官捐献与移植工作将由高速度增长转向高质量发展，坚持以供给侧结构性改革为主线，在积极推动捐献的同时，进一步优化器官移植临床服务质量布局，加强捐献、获取、分配管理力度，规范脑死亡判定流程，加强化解系统性风险的能力，在质的大幅度提升中实现量的有效增长，努力实现更高质量、更有效率、更加公平、可持续的发展。2019 年完成公民逝世后器官捐献 5,818 例，2020 年，即使因受到新冠病毒疫情影响，截至 11 月底我国也仍然实现公民逝世后器官捐献 4,768 例。器官移植医疗质量不断改善，1 年与 5 年存活率已达到世界先进水平，不少器官移植创新技术也开始出现。如：自体肝移植、无缺血器官移植等器官移植技术实现国际领跑；供受者血型不相容肾脏移植技术得到突破；单中心儿童肝移植、心脏移植临床服务能力居世界前列；成立肺移植联盟；器官保存与供体器官维护技术不断改进；肝癌肝移植与乙肝肝移植临床经验已逐步得到国际认可等。经过多年不懈努力，我国器官捐献与移植事业取得快速发展，基本形成了科学公正、遵循伦理、符合我国国情和文化的器官捐献与移植工作模式，并成立了中国人体器官捐献与移植委员会，对器官捐献与移植工作进行顶层设计。目前，我国确定了人体器官捐献与移植工作的基本思路，形成了"政府主导、部门协作、行业推动、社会支持"的工作格局。

2019 年 10 月，党的十九届四中全会明确提出坚持和完善中国特色社会主义制度、推进国家治理体系和治理能力现代化的要求，我们将积极响应党的号召，提高器官移植改革的现代化进程，加强制度建设、体系建设与能力建设，勇敢、坚定地面对挑战，不断完善自己，维护得之不易的改革成果。我们将不懈努力，建设一个完善的并符合伦理和世界卫生组织准则的器官捐献与移植体系，努力攀登器官移植学科相关的科学技术高峰，积极推进"一带一路"器官捐献与移植国际合作，在国际社会展示一个负责任政治大国形象，为建设"人类命运共同体"作出应有的贡献。

本报告记录中国器官移植历史发展新阶段的成绩，将向世界展示中国器官移植改革经验与成果，中国器官移植发展基金会将每年组织编写并出版，实现中英文同时发布。

编 者

2020 年 12 月

Preface

Organ transplantation is a major biomedical development in the 20th century. This technique has gradually matured from clinical experiments to clinical applications and has become an effective medical procedure for treating terminal organ failure. This has saved thousands of patients with organ failure and promoted biomedical science development in China. As organ transplantation requires organs for transplantation from either cadavers or living relatives, it involves social, religious, ethical, political, and legal problems and is intimately associated with a country's traditional culture and socio-economic development.

Organ transplantation needs to take root in China's traditional culture, matches China's state of social development, and comply with globally recognized ethical principles. On March 16, 2006, the former Ministry of Health issued the "Interim Provisions on Clinical Application and Management of Human Organ Transplantation" (Ministry of Health [2006] No. 94) requiring transplantation hospitals to conduct technology access review, unify standards, and stringent management. In the same year, the National Human Organ Transplantation Clinical Application Management Summit was held in Guangzhou and medical staff in the transplantation community reformed the consensus on organ transplantation and issued the "Guangzhou Declaration". This officially heralded the start of reorganization of national organ transplantation medical institutions. The Chinese government pays much attention to the development of human organ donation and transplantation. In May 2007, China's first "Regulations on Human Organ Transplantation" (hereinafter referred to as "regulations" were officially promulgated by the State Council of the People's Republic of China. This symbolizes the gradual improvement in the construction of a human organ donation and transplantation working system in China. In the same year, the former Ministry of Health issued the "Notice of the General Office of the Ministry of Health on the Issues concerning the Application by an Overseas Person for Human Organ Transplantation" (Ministry of Health [2007] No. 11) stipulating the foreign citizens are prohibited from coming to China for organ transplantation tourism. In 2010, the former Ministry of Health and the Red Cross Society of China jointly initiated the "Pilot Program for Organ Donation for Citizens after Death". China's social development stage and traditional culture were used as a basis to establish an organ donation mobilization and witness system in which the Red Cross Society of China is a third-party and international general rules and China's condition were used to propose three types of death judgment criteria for organ donation after citizens have died: Class I (organ donation after brain death); Class II (organ donation after cardiac death); and Class III (organ donation after brain and cardiac death). This laid the theoretical foundation for determining voluntary organ donation after Chinese citizens have died. In 2011, China issued the "Amendment (VIII) to the Criminal Law" that strictly prohibits organ trading and added an "organ trading crime" to further strengthen the legalization of organ donation. In 2011, the China Organ Transplant Response System (COTRS) became operational online. A computer system is used for autonomous allocation with regional priority, critical condition priority, tissue type priority, child priority, matched blood type priority, priority for direct relative of organ donor, rare opportunity priority, waiting sequence priority, and other international organ procurement and allocation principles were complied and an organ donation coordination team was constructed in an orderly manner.

After more than 3 years of efforts, the pilot program achieved success and a more mature work system was developed and a national organ donation management center by the Red Cross Society of China was constructed. On 25 February 2013, the former Ministry of Health and the Red Cross Society of China officially launched voluntary organ donation by citizens after death at the national level. All organ transplantation hospitals must be authorized by the health administrative department to set up organ procurement organizations (OPOs) and organ donation offices. In August 2013, the former National Health and Family Planning Commission promulgated "Human Organ Procurement and Allocation Management Regulations (Interim)", which required all transplantation medical institutions to strictly use COTRS for organ allocation. All institutions, organizations, and individuals are not allowed to allocate donated organs outside of the organ allocation system to ensure that donated human organs are allocated in an open, fair, equal, and traceable manner. In addition, the "Hangzhou Resolution" was announced in the transplantation community. On December 19, 2013, the General Office of the Chinese Communist Party and the General Office of the State Council issued the "Opinions on Party Members and Cadres in Leading Funeral Reform" that encouraged party members and cadres to donate organs and cadavers after death. According to the "Rule of Law" spirit of Fourth Plenary Session of the 18th Central Committee of the Communist Party of China, on December 3, 2014, the National Human Organ Donation and Transplantation Committee officially announced a complete ban in using organs from death row prisoners. This reform received a positive response from the whole of society and recognition from international transplantation societies. As the Chinese saying "It takes 10 years to forge a sword" goes, China has undergone reform to establish 5 major organ donation and transplantation systems (organ donation system, organ procurement and allocation system, organ transplantation medical service system, organ transplantation quality control system, and organ transplantation monitoring system) and has greatly promoted a loving spirit of organ donation in society and a fair, transparent, and cheery atmosphere of voluntary organ donation by citizens has gradually developed in the whole of society.

Health is a common goal of mankind and China's continuous efforts are indispensable to global hygiene and health. Hence, China's hygiene and health also requires support from other countries. In recent years, China has gradually strengthened exchange and collaboration with many countries and comprehensively demonstrated the top-level design, system construction, laws and regulations, and working system of organ transplantation in China.

In addition, China has provided relevant data and analysis results to the international community through the World Health Organization Global Organ Transplantation Monitoring Network and demonstrate China's achievements in human organ donation and transplantation in an open and transparent manner. China's reform has obtained recognition and support from the international community. Since 2006, international organ transplantation experts have provided assistance and guidance to China and jointly published a series of papers on reform with Chinese experts in authoritative international organ transplantation journals. These papers included the "Guangzhou Declaration" in 2006, "Hangzhou Resolution" in 2013, and "Kunming Declaration" in 2019. These experts have witnessed China's organ transplantation reform, and recognized improvements achieved in China's organ transplantation reform in a factual, objective, and fair manner. In August 2016, the 26th International Congress of The Transplantation Society was held in Hong Kong. This is the first Transplantation Society congress held in China, and this is the first time that the congress invited a Chinese expert team to participate in the congress. Professor Jiefu Huang gave the keynote speech during the opening ceremony of the congress and introduced China's 10-year organ transplantation reform process to the world. In October 2016, the China Organ Transplantation Development Foundation and many Chinese and international organ transplantation organizations jointly organized the 1st "China-International Organ Donation Congress" in the Gold Hall of the Great Hall of the People in Beijing. Many experts from institution organ transplantation societies attended the congress and witnessed the official entry of China's organ transplantation into the international community. In February 2017, China was invited to participate in the "Summit on Organ Trafficking and Transplant Tourism" organized by the Pontifical Academy of Sciences. In the face of complex international situation, Chinese representatives factually presented China's voice and narrated China's story, which was widely recognized by leaders from many countries. The "Chinese protocol" for organ donation and transplantation was heralded by the World Health Organization as China's innovation and contribution to transplantation in the world. During the summit,

Professor Francis Delmonico, chairman of the WHO Task Force on Donation and Transplantation of Human Organs and Tissues, mentioned that "Your bones are also our bones, your improvement is also our improvement" and China has gradually integrated into the large international organ transplantation community. Professor José Ramón Núñez, a medical officer in charge of transplantation at World Health Organization once said that "China wasn't on the ship of world organ transplantation, and we had no idea where it headed. But after 2015, China has been standing in the center of the ship." In March 2018, a declaration on China's organ transplantation reform experience was released during the "Ethics in Action" meeting jointly organized by the United Nations and the Pontifical Academy of Sciences. In the meeting, the "Pontifical Academy of Sciences Ethics in Action meeting declaration" mentioned that "The basic characteristics of the China model are demonstrated by the determination of the Chinese government in continuous reform and cooperation between transplantation experts led by Professor Jiefu Huang and the government: in efficient implementation of organ transplantation reform measures". In May 2018, China participated in the 71st World Health Assembly and 100 transplantation experts from China attended the meeting and introduced China's reform experience. The Director-General of the World Health Organization, Dr. Tedros Adhanom praised and thanked China for its contributions to world transplantation. In August 2018, the WHO Task Force on Donation and Transplantation of Human Organs and Tissues that China suggested to set up was officially formed at the 27th International Congress of The Transplantation Society, which was held in Madrid, Spain. 31 experts form this task force, of which 2 were from China. Jiefu Huang was nominated as a World Health Organization transplantation consultant and China has started contributing its knowledge for global governance of transplantation.

In recent years, China has successively promulgated and established regulations and systems for organ donation. For example, in 2016, 6 national departments such as the Ministry of Transport, Civil Aviation Administration, and National Railway Administration jointly set up a green channel for organ transportation to gain precious time to save lives. In May 2017, the "Law of the People's Republic of China on the Red Cross Society" was revised to clearly promote organ donation and explore charity organizations and other humanitarian relief mechanisms. The quantity and quality of organ donations and transplantations in China is undergoing rapid development. From 2015 to 2018, the number of organ donations increased continuously at a rate of 22%-47.5%. In 2015, 2016, 2017, and 2018, the number of deceased organ donations was 2766, 4080, 5146, and 6302, respectively. In addition, there were 2200-2500 living relative donations every year. In 2018, 20201 organ transplantation surgeries were carried out, which was ranked second globally. In 2019, the National Health Commission mentioned that China's organ donation and transplantation work will transition from rapid increase to high quality development and mainly focus on structural reform at the supply end. While aggressively promoting organ donation, organ transplantation clinical service quality layout will be further optimized; donation, procurement, and allocation management will be strengthened; the procedure for determining brain death will be regulated; and capabilities in reducing systematic risk will be strengthened to achieve effective growth in quantity while increasing quality. This will enable high quality, more efficient, fairer, and sustainable development. In 2019, 5813 deceased organ donations were completed. Up till November 2020, 4768 deceased organ donations were completed even though coronavirus disease 2019 affected donation. Organ transplantation medicine quality has continuously improved and the 1-year and 5-year survival rates have reached global advanced levels and many innovative organ transplantation techniques have emerged. Examples include: liver auto transplantation and non-ischemic organ transplantation, which China is leading internationally. Breakthroughs were also achieved in incompatible blood type renal transplantation. China's single-center pediatric liver transplantation and heart transplantation clinical services are also top in the world. China has also established a liver transplantation alliance and has made continuous improvements in organ storage and donor organ maintenance techniques. China's clinical experience in liver cancer liver transplantation and hepatitis B liver transplantation have also gradually received international recognition.

After many years of efforts, active progress was made in China's organ donation and transplantation industry to basically form an organ donation and transplantation working model that is scientific and fair, complies with ethics, and in line with China's condition and culture. The China National Organ Donation and Transplantation Committee was set up for top-level design. The committee confirm the basic thought processes for human organ donation and transplantation work and established a "government-led, department-coordinated, industry-promoted, and society-supported" working model.

On October 2019, the Fourth Plenary Session of the 19th Central Committee of the Communist Party of China proposed to maintain and improve China's system of socialist characteristics and promote modernization of the national governance system and governance capabilities. We will actively heed the call of the party, improve modernization in organ transplantation reform, strengthen system and capacity building, face challenges in a bold and steadfast manner, and continuously improve ourselves to protect reform achievements that were not easily obtained. We will strive to establish a complete organ donation and transplantation system that complies with ethics and World Health Organization principles, strive to reach the science and technology peak in organ transplantation medicine, actively promote "Belt and Road Initiative" international collaboration in organ donation and transplantation, and demonstrate a responsible major political country to the international community, and contribute to establishing a "Community with shared future for mankind".

This report records the achievements in the new phase of China's organ transplantation history and development to demonstrate China's organ transplantation reform experience to the world. Every year, the China Organ Transplantation Development Foundation will draft new editions and both English and Chinese versions will be simultaneously released.

Editorial Committee
December, 2020

目　录

Contents

第一章　中国人体器官分配与共享

本章内容为基于中国人体器官分配与共享计算机系统（China Organ Transplant Response System，COTRS）的数据分析，统计范围是中国内地，不包含港澳台地区。

自 2015 年 1 月 1 日至 2019 年 12 月 31 日，中国公民逝世后器官捐献（Deceased Donation, DD）累计完成 24,112 例。2019 年中国完成公民逝世后器官捐献 5,818 例，器官移植手术 19,454 例。每百万人口器官捐献率（permillion population，PMP）从 2015 年的 2.01 上升至 2019 年的 4.16。

中国人体器官捐献和移植的五大工作体系包括：人体器官捐献体系、人体器官获取与分配体系、人体器官移植临床服务体系、人体器官移植质控体系和人体器官捐献与移植监管体系（图 1-1）。目前，中国已实现了科学、公平、公正的器官分配。

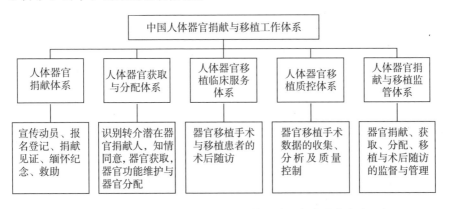

图 1-1　中国人体器官捐献与移植工作体系（不包含港澳台地区）

COTRS 是我国器官捐献与移植工作体系的重要组成部分，由"潜在器官捐献者识别系统""人体器官捐献人登记及器官匹配系统"以及"人体器官移植等待者预约名单系统" 3 个子系统以及监管平台组成。

COTRS 是《人体器官移植条例》第六条、第二十二条规定和国家《刑法修正案（八）》第二百三十四条等有关器官移植和捐献法律条款的重要体现和落实。2018 年国家卫生健康委印发了《关于印发中国人体器官分配与共享基本原则和核心政策的通知》（国卫医发〔2018〕24 号），对《卫生部关于印发中国人体器官分配与共享基本原则和肝脏与肾脏移植核心政策的通知》（卫医管发〔2010〕113 号）进行了修订，并制定了心脏、肺脏分配与共享核心政策，形成了《中国人体器官分配与共享基本原则和核心政策》。

一方面，作为执行我国器官分配与共享相关法律法规和科学政策的高度专用的关键系统。COTRS 执行国家器官科学分配政策，实施自动器官分配和共享，并向国家和地方监管机构提供全程监控，建立器官获取和分配的溯源性，最大限度地排除人为干预，保障器官分配的公平、公正、公开，是我国公民逝世后器官捐献工作赢得人民群众信任的重要基石。另一方面，COTRS 已通过国家信息安全测评中心认证，并采用权限控制及监控相关医疗机构操作等方式，确保捐受双方及器官分配过程中的信息安全，保障患者隐私。

一、器官捐献与移植医疗资源分布

1. 全国器官获取组织分布

我国人体器官捐献与移植体系中，器官获取组织（Organ Procurement Organization, OPO）是以医疗机构为单位，设立器官捐献与获取专业团队。该团队由医务人员、器官捐献协调员、行政管理人员等组成。这一点与美国的 OPO 和西班牙的国家器官移植组织（Organization National De Transplantz, ONT）有所不同。

截至 2019 年 12 月 31 日，除港澳台外，全中国共有 125 个 OPO，各省（区、市）OPO 数量分布见图 1-2。

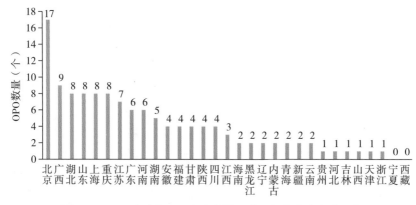

图 1-2　2019 年中国 OPO 分布情况（不包含港澳台地区）

2. 全国移植中心分布

截至 2019 年 12 月 31 日，除港澳台外，全国具有 173 所器官移植资质的医疗机构，各省（区、市）移植医疗机构分布见图 1-3。其中，数量排名居前五位的省（区、市）为广东（19）、北京（17）、山东（13）、上海（11）、湖南（9）和浙江（9）。

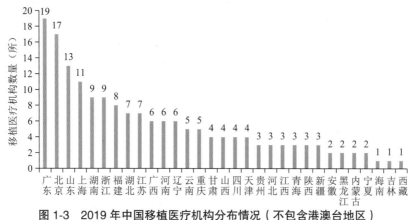

图 1-3　2019 年中国移植医疗机构分布情况（不包含港澳台地区）

二、人体器官捐献情况

1. 人体器官捐献情况

2015 年至 2019 年，我国公民逝世后器官捐献量分别为 2,766 例、4,080

例、5,146 例、6,302 例和 5,818 例，PMP 分别为 2.01、2.98、3.72、4.53、4.16（图 1-4）。

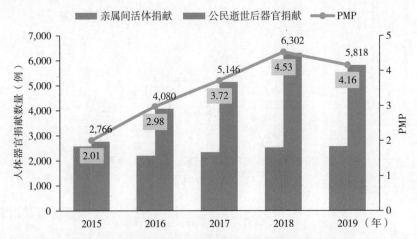

图 1-4　2015—2019 年中国人体器官捐献量（不包含港澳台地区）

注：2015—2017 年人口数来自《中国卫生健康统计年鉴》。

2015 年至 2019 年逝世后器官捐献量居前五位的省（区、市）为：广东（3,290）、湖北（2,472）、山东（2,428）、湖南（2,126）和北京（1,898）。2015 年至 2019 年各省（区、市）捐献量分布见图 1-5。

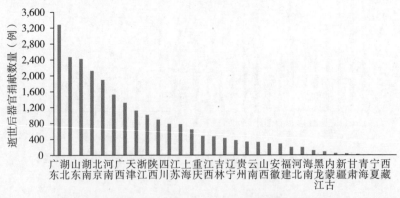

图 1-5　2015—2019 年中国各省（区、市）逝世后器官捐献量（不包含港澳台地区）

2019 年逝世后器官捐献量排名前五位的省（区、市）为：广东（890）、湖北（599）、山东（495）、天津（457）和湖南（429）。青海实现人体器官捐献量零的突破。

12个省（区、市）PMP超过全国水平（4.16），PMP排名前五位的省（区、市）为：天津（29.29）、北京（13.79）、湖北（10.12）、广东（7.84）和海南（7.60）。2019年各省（区、市）PMP分布见图1-6。

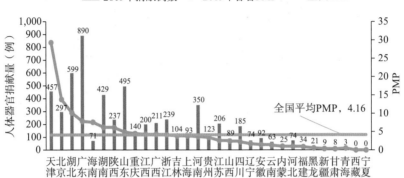

图 1-6　2019 年中国逝世后器官捐献量与 PMP（不包含港澳台地区）

2015年至2019年，5年间全国有10个OPO完成逝世后器官捐献600例以上，有10个OPO完成捐献300～600例，有15个OPO完成捐献200～299例。其中，2019年全国3个OPO完成捐献200例以上，有10个OPO完成捐献100～200例，有23个OPO完成捐献50～99例。

2. 器官捐献者特征

2019年，中国公民逝世后捐献者年龄中位数为47岁，儿童捐献者（18岁以下）占8.20%。捐献者性别以男性为主，占比为81.57%。捐献者的血型以O型为主，占38.12%；其次是A型和B型，分别占28.45%和25.95%；AB型占7.48%（图1-7）。32.76%为中国Ⅰ类（脑死亡器官捐献），44.35%为中国Ⅱ类（心脏死亡器官捐献），22.89%为中国Ⅲ类（心—脑双死亡器官捐献）（图1-8）。

2015年至2019年，创伤和脑血管意外为逝世后器官捐献者两大主要死亡原因，占所有死亡原因的86.82%（图1-9）。其中，脑血管意外死亡的捐献者占比逐年上升。2019年，脑血管意外超过创伤，成为中国公民逝世后器官捐献的主要死亡原因（图1-10）。

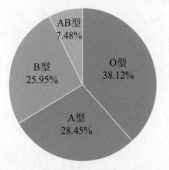

图 1-7 2019 年中国公民逝世后器官捐献者血型分布（不包含港澳台地区）

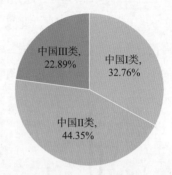

图 1-8 2019 年中国公民逝世后器官捐献者中国分类（不包含港澳台地区）

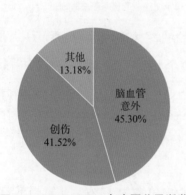

图 1-9 2015—2019 年中国公民逝世后器官捐献者死亡原因（不包含港澳台地区）

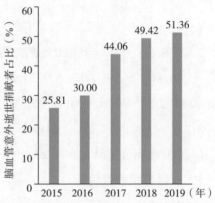

图 1-10 2015—2019 年中国公民脑血管意外逝世捐献者占比 (%)（不包含港澳台地区）

三、移植等待者情况

2015 年至 2019 年，肝肾器官移植等待者数量（图 1-11）逐年增加；2017 年至 2019 年每年肝脏移植器官等待者数量明显高于 2015 年和 2016。截至 2019 年年底，全国仍有 47,382 人等待肾脏移植、4,763 人等待肝脏移植。心脏、肺脏分配系统于 2018 年 10 月 22 日启用，2019 年年底，仍有 338 人等待心脏移植，89 人等待肺脏移植。

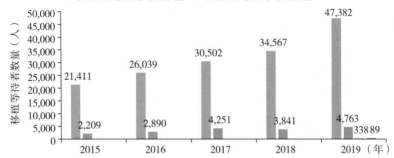

图 1-11　2015—2019 年历年年末器官移植等待者数量（不包含港澳台地区）

除港澳台地区外，2019 年全国各省（区、市）肾脏移植等待者数量分布见图 1-12，其中排名前五位省（区、市）分别为：广东（6,105）、浙江（5,155）、湖南（4,937）、四川（3,724）和上海（3,644）

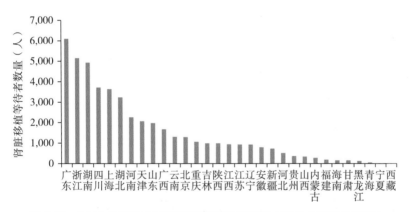

图 1-12　2019 年年底中国肾脏移植等待者数量（不包含港澳台地区）

2019 年年底，除港澳台地区外，全国各省（区、市）肝脏移植等待者数量分布见图 1-13，其中排名前五位的省（区、市）分别为：四川（1,142）、广东（805）、天津（558）、上海（372）和北京（298）。

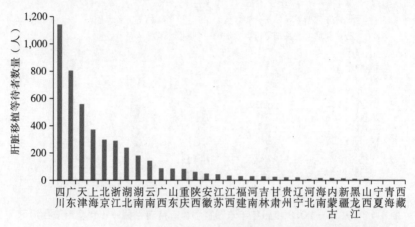

图 1-13　2019 年年底中国肝脏移植等待者数量（不包含港澳台地区）

2019 年年底，除港澳台地区外，全国各省（区、市）心脏移植等待者数量分布见图 1-14，其中排名前五位的省（区、市）分别为：北京（108）、广东（37）、湖北（30）、上海（25）和浙江（23）。

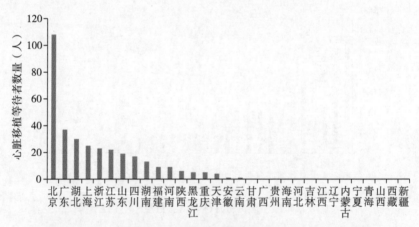

图 1-14　2019 年年底中国心脏移植等待者数量（不包含港澳台地区）

2019 年年底，除港澳台地区外，全国各省（区、市）肺脏移植等待者数量分布见图 1-15，其中排名前五位的省（区、市）分别为：广东（21）、江苏（13）、湖北（12）、上海（10）和浙江（9）。

8

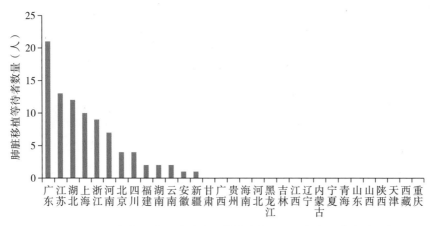

图 1-15　2019 年年底中国肺脏移植等待者数量（不包含港澳台地区）

四、器官利用情况

1. 逝世后器官捐献者产出器官情况

2015 年至 2019 年，每位逝世后捐献者平均产出的肾脏器官数分别为 1.92、1.87、1.89、1.91 和 1.89 个，平均年产出的肝脏器官数分别为 0.88、0.87、0.90、0.91 和 0.93 个（图 1-16）。2019 年，每位捐献者平均产出的心脏器官数为 0.12 个，平均年产出的肺脏器官数为 0.15 个。

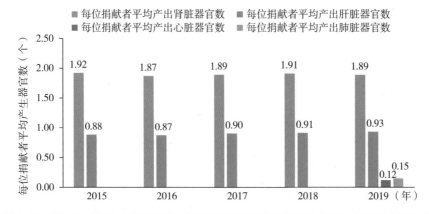

图 1-16　2015—2019 年每位逝世后器官捐献者产出的器官数（不包含港澳台地区）

2. 绿色通道政策实施前后器官共享对比

原国家卫生和计划生育委员会、公安部、交通运输部、中国民用航空局、中国铁路总公司、中国红十字会总会于 2016 年 5 月 6 日联合印发了《关于建立人体捐献器官转运绿色通道的通知》（以下简称《通知》），建立人体捐献器官转运绿色通道。《通知》明确了各方职责，目的是确保人体捐献器官转运流程的通畅，将器官转运环节对器官移植患者的质量安全影响减少到最低程度。

《通知》将器官转运分为一般流程及应急流程，转运过程中根据实际情况启动不同流程，实现人体捐献器官转运的快速通关与优先承运，提高转运效率，保障转运安全，减少因运输原因造成的器官浪费。

比较人体捐献器官转运绿色通道政策实施前后全国人体器官共享情况，结果显示，政策实施后器官全国共享比例总体上升 7.8%，其中肾脏全国共享比例上升了 5.9%，肝脏全国共享比例上升了 6.4%（表 1-1）。

表 1-1　绿色通道政策实施前后全国肝肾器官共享率（%）（不包含港澳台地区）

时间段	总体共享率（%）			肾脏共享率（%）			肝脏共享率（%）		
	政策前	政策后	变化	政策前	政策后	变化	政策前	政策后	变化
中心自用	75.0	66.5	−8.5	84.6	77.6	−7.0	53.2	48.7	−4.5
省内共享	12.6	13.3	0.7 ▲	10.5	11.6	1.1 ▲	17.3	15.4	−1.9
全国共享	12.4	20.2	7.8 ▲	4.9	10.8	5.9 ▲	29.5	35.9	6.4 ▲

五、特点与展望

器官移植是人类医学发展的巨大成就，挽救了无数终末期疾病患者的生命。2019 年中国器官捐献、移植数量均位居世界第二位。

1. 进一步提高捐献器官利用率

我国人口众多，患者数量庞大，器官短缺依旧是制约器官移植事业发展的主要原因之一。在捐献器官短缺的情况下，应加强供体器官功能维护、扩大器官供给，进一步提升心脏、肺脏移植医疗技术，提高器官利用率。

此外，应扩大器官捐献方面的宣传教育，提高公众对器官捐献工作的认知。

2. 进一步发挥绿色通道作用，减少器官转运的浪费

随着我国器官捐献工作的进一步推进，捐献器官全国匹配共享的数量越来越多。器官转运绿色通道政策实现人体捐献器官转运的快速通关与优先承运、提高转运效率、保障转运安全、减少在器官运输过程中造成的器官浪费。

3. 推动器官捐献与移植事业由高速度增长向高质量发展

近年来我国器官捐献、移植的数量和质量都在不断提升。伴随医疗卫生条件的改善和人民群众对医疗健康期望的提高，人民群众对移植服务的需求与移植事业发展不平衡、不充分仍存在巨大矛盾。

我们在注重发展数量和速度的同时，更要推动器官捐献与移植事业由高速度增长向高质量发展。在积极推动捐献的同时，进一步优化器官移植临床服务资源布局，着力解决区域之间、学科之间器官移植技术能力发展不平衡的问题，加强捐献、获取、分配管理力度。在质的大幅度提升中实现量的持续健康增长，努力实现更高质量、更高效率、更加公平的可持续发展。

第二章 中国肝脏移植

本章内容主要基于中国肝脏移植注册系统（China Liver Transplant Registry, CLTR）的数据分析。数据统计范围为中国内地数据，不包含港澳台地区。

CLTR 是在国家卫生健康委督导下建立的国家官方肝脏移植注册系统，要求全国具有肝脏移植资质的医疗机构必须及时、完整地向其填报移植相关信息。CLTR 通过对中国内地的肝脏移植情况进行动态、科学地分析，描述肝脏移植专业医疗质量现状，为国家监管部门制定移植相关的政策、法规提供了依据，也为各移植中心提供了肝脏移植受者的科学管理工具。迄今为止，CLTR 已成为中国器官移植领域最重要的信息化系统以及肝脏移植学术交流平台之一。

一、肝脏移植医疗机构分布

截至 2019 年 12 月 31 日，全国共有 105 所具有肝脏移植资质的医疗机构。其中，肝脏移植医疗机构数量较集中的省（区、市）为北京（12）、广东（12）、上海（9）、山东（8）和浙江（6）（图 2-1）

2015 年至 2019 年，全国共实施肝脏移植 23,890 例，包括公民逝世后器官捐献肝脏移植（ deceased donor liver transplantation, DDLT）20,630 例，占比 86.4%；亲属间活体肝脏移植（ living-related donor liver transplantation, LDLT）3,260 例，占比 13.6%。成人肝脏移植 19,760 例，占比 82.7%；儿童肝脏移植 4,130 例，占比 17.3%。

2019 年，全国共实施肝脏移植手术 6,170 例，包括 5,332 例 DDLT，占比86.4%；838例LDLT（包括7例多米诺肝脏移植），占比13.6%。成人肝脏移植5,075例，占比82.3%；儿童肝脏移植1,095例，占比17.7%。2019年实施肝脏移植例数排名前5位的省（区、市）依次为上海（1,267）、广东（664）、北京（605）、天津（602）、浙江（586）；2019年实施100例以上肝脏移植的省（区、市）有14个，移植总量占全国当年总例数的92.4%（图2-2）；内蒙古、宁夏在2019年度未开展肝脏移植（西藏暂无具有肝脏移植资质的医疗机构）。

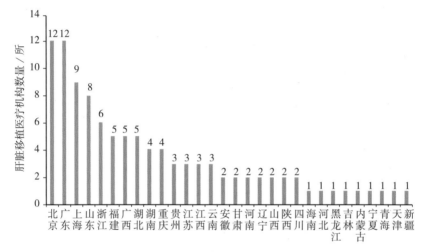

图2-1　2019年中国具有肝脏移植资质的医疗机构分布（不包含港澳台地区）

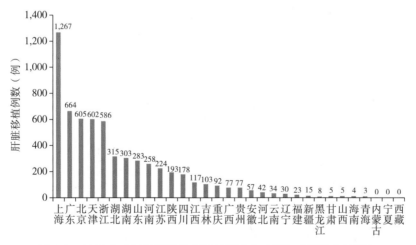

图2-2　2019年中国肝脏移植例数地区分布（不包含港澳台地区）

2019 年有 10 所医疗机构实施的肝脏移植例数在 200 例及以上，其移植总量占全国当年总例数的 50.6%（表 2-1）。

表 2-1　2019 年中国肝脏移植例数排名前十位的医疗机构（不包含港澳台地区）

地 区	肝脏移植医疗机构	例数
上海	上海交通大学医学院附属仁济医院	688
天津	天津市第一中心医院	602
浙江	浙江大学医学院附属第一医院	280
广东	中山大学附属第三医院	252
上海	复旦大学附属中山医院	244
上海	复旦大学附属华山医院	226
浙江	树兰（杭州）医院	221
河南	郑州大学第一附属医院	208
湖南	中南大学湘雅二医院	201
北京	首都医科大学附属北京友谊医院	200

二、肝脏移植受者人口特征

2019 年我国肝脏移植受者的年龄均值 42.2 岁，中位数 48.7 岁；受者体质指数（Body Mass Index, BMI）均值 22.3kg/m²，中位数 22.5 kg/m²；以男性受者为主，占比 75.0%；受者血型以 O 型、A 型、B 型为主，且三种血型的受者各占 30% 左右，血型为 AB 型的受者占比最少（表 2-2）。

表 2-2　2019 年中国肝脏移植受者人口特征（不包含港澳台地区）

变量	均值 ± 标准差	占比（%）
年龄（岁）	42.2 ± 20.8	--
BMI（kg/ ㎡）	22.3 ± 4.4	--
性别		
男	--	75.0
女	--	25.0
血型		
O 型	--	30.2
A 型	--	30.5
B 型	--	29.0
AB 型	--	10.3

三、肝脏移植质量安全分析

1. 肝脏移植重要临床指标

2019年,我国LDLT的平均冷缺血时间、平均无肝期、术中平均失血量、术中平均输红细胞(Red Blood Cell, RBC)量均低于 DDLT,LDLT 的平均手术时间略高于 DDLT(图 2-3 至图 2-7)。

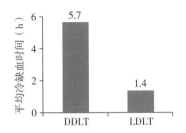

图 2-3 2019 年肝脏移植平均冷缺血时间(不包含港澳台地区)

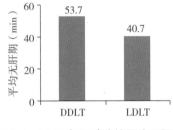

图 2-4 2019 年肝脏移植平均无肝期(不包含港澳台地区)

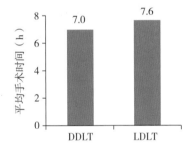

图 2-5 2019 年肝脏移植平均手术时间(不包含港澳台地区)

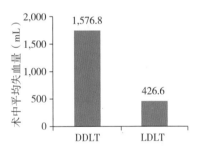

图 2-6 2019 年肝脏移植术中平均失血量(不包含港澳台地区)

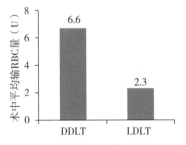

图 2-7 2019 年肝脏移植术中平均输 RBC 量(不包含港澳台地区)

2. 肝脏移植前后受者总胆红素的变化情况

分别对 2019 年 DDLT 受者和 LDLT 受者术前、术后各时间点的总胆红素变化情况进行分析,移植受者术后总胆红素平均值呈明显下降趋势(表 2-3)。

表 2-3　2019 年肝脏移植受者术前、术后的总胆红素平均值(不包含港澳台地区)

时间	总胆红素平均值(μmol/L)	
	DDLT	LDLT
术前	214.1	227.5
术后 1 周	62.3	48.3
术后 2 周	45.3	25.6
术后 1 个月	30.6	17.7
术后 3 个月	20.4	11.8
术后 6 个月	21.0	12.4

3. 肝脏移植受者术后情况

(1)术后 30 天内并发症

2019 年,我国 DDLT 受者术后 30 天内并发症发生率为 33.9%,主要为胸腔积液(19.7%)、术后感染(15.4%)、腹腔内积液或脓肿(12.9%);LDLT 受者术后 30 天内并发症发生率为 16.5%,主要为术后感染(8.1%)、腹腔内积液或脓肿(5.4%)、胸腔积液(3.7%)。

(2)术后 30 天内死亡率

2019 年,我国 DDLT 受者术后 30 天内死亡率为 5.3%;LDLT 受者术后 30 天内死亡率为 2.7%。

(3)肝脏移植术后受者、移植物生存情况

选取 2015 年至 2019 年期间全国范围内开展的肝脏移植病例进行受者和移植物的生存分析,结果如下:

我国 DDLT 受者术后 1 年、3 年累计生存率分别为 83.3%、74.4%;LDLT 受者术后 1 年、3 年累计生存率分别为 91.8%、88.5%。

我国 DDLT 移植物术后 1 年、3 年累计生存率分别为 82.5%、73.2%;LDLT 移植物术后 1 年、3 年累计生存率分别为 91.3%、87.5%(表

2-4）。

表 2-4 2015—2019 年中国肝脏移植受者/移植物术后生存率（不包含港澳台地区）

分组	术后 1 年生存率（%）		术后 3 年生存率（%）	
	受者	移植物	受者	移植物
DDLT	83.3	82.5	74.4	73.2
LDLT	91.8	91.3	88.5	87.5

（4）肝癌肝脏移植受者术后无瘤生存情况

2015 年至 2019 年，我国肝癌肝脏移植受者术后 1 年、3 年无瘤生存率分别为 77.6%、62.5%。

四、特点与展望

近年来，中国肝脏移植的数量和质量稳步提升，跻身国际前列。2019 年全国肝脏移植例数继续保持在 6,000 例以上。

1. 儿童肝脏移植发展迅速

2019 年中国儿童肝脏移植占比 17.7%。我国年实施儿童肝脏移植例数最多的上海交通大学医学院附属仁济医院在 2019 年实施儿童肝脏移植 443 例。

2. 亲属间活体肝脏移植占比较高

2019 年，我国亲属间活体肝脏移植占比为 13.6%，达到 838 例。在我国儿童肝脏移植中，亲属间活体来源占 70.4%，反映出我国亲属间更加紧密的关系纽带。

3. 原发病是肝癌的肝脏移植比例较高

我国是肝癌高发国家，2019 年在 DDLT 受者中，恶性肿瘤比例为 42.1%。我国提出的肝癌肝脏移植杭州标准得到了学术界的广泛认可和临床应用，可在扩大肝癌肝脏移植受者入选范围的同时，保持其生存率与国际水平无明显差异。

4. 不断探索肝脏移植手术方式和技术

实现肝脏移植吻合方式的变革，吻合部位从胃十二指肠动脉改为脾动脉，显著改善术后肝脏血流，降低胆道并发症等的发生率；开展无缺血肝脏移植；实施两人互换部分肝脏交叉辅助多米诺肝脏移植手术，为两个患有不同遗传代谢缺陷肝病的患者互换半个肝脏，实现了不需要器官捐献的器官移植等。

5. 建立并落实肝脏移植医疗质量管理与控制有关规范和制度

进一步完善捐献肝脏质量维护与评估体系，提高捐献肝脏质量，降低并发症的发生率，提高受者生存率；加强术后重要并发症的监测，如术后早期肝功能不全（EAD）、急性肾损伤（AKI）、新发糖尿病等质控指标；以更加科学化、精细化的质控体系，实现全国肝脏移植临床质量、服务和疗效的提升。

6. 科学监管肝脏移植数据，挖掘有价值的信息

加强信息化建设，利用大数据思维和精细化管理开展临床研究，利用循证医学证据指导临床决策；汇聚临床优势资源，创新引领肝脏移植领域多中心高质量的临床研究，推进科研成果临床转化与应用，推动肝脏移植学科发展。

第三章 中国肾脏移植

本章内容主要基于中国肾脏移植科学登记系统（Chinese Scientific Registry of Kidney Transplantation，CSRKT）的数据分析。数据统计范围是中国内地数据，不包含港澳台地区。

CSRKT 是在国家卫生健康委督导下建立的、具有官方性质的肾脏移植注册系统，要求全国具有肾脏移植资质的医疗机构必须及时、完整地向其填报移植相关信息。CSRKT 作为中国唯一的肾脏移植受者科学登记系统，通过对中国内地的肾脏移植情况进行动态、科学地分析，为国家监管部门制定移植相关的政策、法规提供了依据，也为各移植中心提供了肾脏移植受者的科学管理工具。迄今为止，CSRKT 已成为中国器官移植领域最重要的信息化系统以及肾脏移植学术交流平台之一。

一、肾脏移植医疗机构分布

截至 2019 年 12 月 31 日，中国共有 135 所医疗机构被授予肾脏移植开展资质，医疗机构分布较多的省（区、市）为广东（18）、北京（13）、山东（11）、湖南（9）、浙江（8）等（图 3-1）。

2015 年至 2019 年，中国共实施肾脏移植 52,005 例，其中 DD 肾脏移植（deceased donor kidney transplantation）42,886 例，亲属间活体肾脏移植（living-related donor kidney transplantation）9,119 例。2019 年实施肾脏移植 12,124 例，其中 DD 肾脏移植 10,389 例，较 2018 年减少 8.1%；亲属间活体肾脏移植 1,735 例，较 2018 年减少 6.9%（图 3-2）。

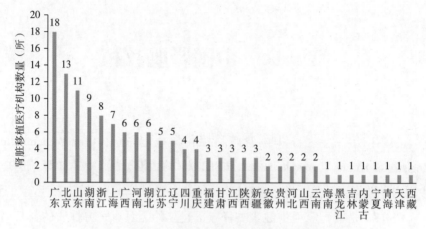

图 3-1　中国具有肾脏移植资质的医疗机构地理分布

（截至 2019 年年底，不包含港澳台地区）

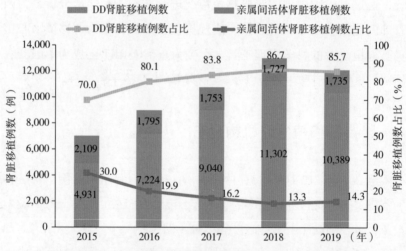

图 3-2　2015—2019 年中国肾脏移植实施例数（不包含港澳台地区）

　　2019 年中国共实施肾脏相关的多器官联合移植 224 例，其中肝肾联合移植 68 例、胰肾联合移植 149 例、心肾联合移植 7 例。较 2018 年增加 45.5%（图 3-3）。

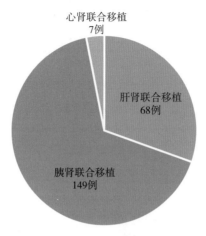

图 3-3 2019 年中国肾脏相关的多器官联合移植实施例数（不包含港澳台地区）

2019 年实施肾脏相关的多器官联合移植例数排名前五位的省（区、市）是天津（69）、广东（66）、湖南 (16)、广西 (15) 和山东 (12)（图 3-4），表 3-1 为排名前十位的医疗机构情况。

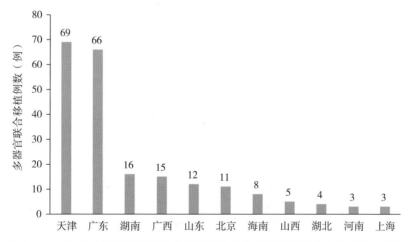

图 3-4 2019 年中国肾脏相关的多器官联合移植实施例数前十名省（区、市）
（不包含港澳台地区）

表 3-1 2019 年中国肾脏相关的多器官联合移植实施例数前十名医疗机构
（不包含港澳台地区）

地区	肾脏移植医院	例数
天津	天津市第一中心医院	69
广东	广州医科大学附属第二医院	54
湖南	郴州市第一人民医院	13
广西	解放军联勤保障部队第九二三医院	11
山东	青岛大学附属医院	10
北京	解放军总医院	9
海南	海南医学院第二附属医院	8
广东	中山大学附属第一医院	7
山西	山西省第二人民医院	5
湖北	华中科技大学同济医学院附属同济医院	3

儿童（＜18 岁）肾脏移植近年来得到广泛关注，2019 年儿童肾脏移植例数占全国总例数的 2.9%（图 3-5）。

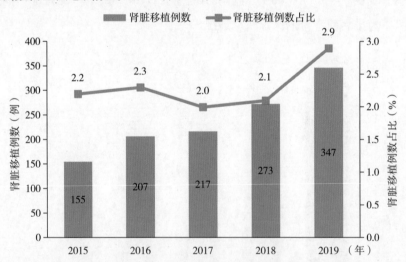

图 3-5 2015—2019 年中国儿童肾脏移植实施例数及占比（不包含港澳台地区）

2019 年实施肾脏移植例数排名前五位的省（区、市）是：广东（1,769）、湖北（1,318）、山东（965）、浙江（924）和湖南（897），各省（区、市）实施的肾脏移植例数分布见图 3-6。

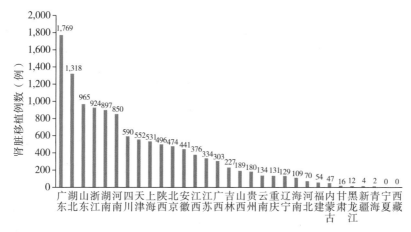

图 3-6　2019 年中国各省（区、市）肾脏移植例数分布（不包含港澳台地区）

2019 年实施肾脏移植 ≥ 250 例的医疗机构有 14 所，其实施的肾脏移植例数占比当年总例数的 44.4%；此外 200～249 例的有 5 所，100～199 例的有 19 所，50～99 例的有 25 所，10～49 例的有 40 所，1～9 例的有 19 所，有 13 所未开展肾脏移植（其中 8 所在 2017 年至 2019 年连续 3 年未开展肾脏移植）。2019 年各数量区间的肾脏移植例数及中国总例数占比见表 3-2。

表 3-2　2019 年中国肾脏移植数量区间分布及占比（不包含港澳台地区）

例数区间	医疗机构数	例数占比（%）
≥ 250	14	44.4
200～249	5	9.1
100～199	19	21.9
50～99	25	14.7
10～49	40	9.3
1～9	19	0.6
0	13	0

2019 年中国肾脏移植手术的开展具有较为明显的区域优势特征，有 6 个省（区、市）实施肾脏移植 ≥ 600 例，占全国当年总例数的 55.5%（表 3-3）。

表 3-3　2019 年中国各省（区、市）肾脏移植例数分布（不包含港澳台地区）

例数区间	医疗机构数	例数占比（%）
≥ 600	6	55.5
400 ~ 599	6	25.4
200 ~ 399	4	10.2
100 ~ 199	6	7.2
1 ~ 99	7	1.7
0	2	0

　　2019 年中国 DD 肾脏移植例数前十位的省（区、市）是广东（1,713）、湖北（1,264）、湖南（834）、山东（820）、浙江（708）、河南（678）、天津（517）、上海（468）、陕西（442）、北京（394），共占当年中国 DD 总例数的 75.4%（图 3-7）。

　　2019 年亲属间活体肾脏移植实施例数位居前五位的省（区、市）是四川（295）、安徽（290）、浙江（216）、河南（172）、山东（145）（图 3-8）。

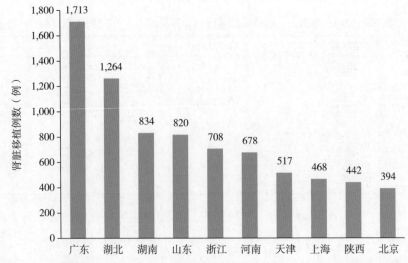

图 3-7　2019 年中国 DD 肾脏移植实施例数前十名省（区、市）（不包含港澳台地区）

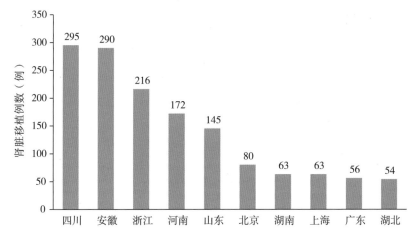

图 3-8 2019 年中国亲属间活体肾脏移植例数前十名省（区、市）（不包含港澳台地区）

二、肾脏移植受者人口特征

对 2019 年中国内地实施的肾脏移植病例数据分析，结果显示：受者年龄为（40.1±12.1）岁，BMI 为（23.1±4.3）kg/m²，术前透析时间为（771±876）天，男性移植受者占比 70.6%，AB 血型移植受者占比最少为 9.0%（表 3-4）。

表 3-4 2019 年中国肾脏移植受者人口特征（不包含港澳台地区）

变量	均数 ± 标准差
受者年龄（岁）	40.1 ± 12.1
BMI（kg/m²）	23.1 ± 4.3
术前透析时间（天）	771 ± 876
受者血型	占比（%）
O 型	34.2
A 型	30.0
B 型	26.8
AB 型	9.0
性别	占比（%）
男	70.6
女	29.4

（1）儿童肾脏移植受者（＜18岁）347例，占比2.9%；（18～30）岁的受者2,062例，占17.0%；（30～50）岁的受者6,792例，占56.0%；（50～65）岁的受者2,723例，占22.5%；老年肾脏移植≥65岁以上受者200例，占1.6%。

（2）儿童捐献者（＜18岁）占比7.7%，其中＜1岁的捐献者占比15.0%、（1～7）岁的捐献者占比35.5%、（7～12）岁的捐献者占比20.6%、（12～18）岁的捐献者占比28.9%。

三、肾脏移植质量安全分析

1. DD肾脏移植供肾缺血时间

分别对2019年亲属间活体、DD肾脏移植病例进行分析，供肾平均冷缺血时间不超过6小时（表3-5）。99%的亲属间活体和98.5%的DD肾脏移植的供肾冷缺血时间≤24小时；98.1%的亲属间活体和81.3%的DD肾脏移植的供肾热缺血时间≤10分钟（表3-6）。

表3-5　2019年亲属间活体、DD肾脏移植供肾缺血时间（不包含港澳台地区）

变量	亲属间活体（均值±标准差）	DD（均值±标准差）
供肾冷缺血时间（小时）	1.9±1.3	5.8±3.8
供肾热缺血时间（分钟）	3.7±3.3	8.7±7.4

表3-6　2019年亲属间活体、DD肾脏移植供肾缺血时间占比（不包含港澳台地区）

变量	亲属间活体（%）	DD（%）
供肾冷缺血时间≤24（小时）	99.0	98.5
供肾热缺血时间≤10（分钟）	98.1	81.3

2. 肾脏移植前后受者血清肌酐值的变化情况

2019年全国共实施12,124例肾脏移植手术，根据CSRKT要求，分析4个随访时间点（术前、术后30天、术后180天、术后360天）的亲属间活体肾脏移植、DD肾脏移植受者的血清肌酐平均值（表3-7）。

表 3-7 2019 年亲属间活体、DD 肾脏移植受者术前与术后的血清肌酐平均值
（不包含港澳台地区）

时间点	亲属间活体（μmol/L）	DD（μmol/L）
术前	986.7	914.2
术后 30 天	119.4	150.0
术后 180 天	115.0	123.5
术后 360 天	119.5	115.6

3. 肾脏移植术后不良事件概况

肾脏移植术后不良事件主要包括：移植肾功能延迟恢复、急性排斥反应、感染、移植受者死亡、移植肾丢失等。对 2019 年病例的随访资料进行分析，主要不良事件发生率见表 3-8、表 3-9。术后 30 天内死亡率为 0.4%。未见亲属间活体捐献者术后 30 天内有重大并发症发生者。

表 3-8 2019 年中国肾脏移植术后不良事件发生率（不包含港澳台地区）

不良事件	亲属间活体（%）	DD（%）
移植肾功能延迟恢复	1.3	8.7
急性排斥反应	3.2	3.1
感染	3.7	5.9
移植受者死亡	0.5	1.2
移植肾全因丢失	1.2	4.3

表 3-9 2019 年中国胰肾联合移植术后不良事件发生率（不包含港澳台地区）

不良事件	总体发生率（%）
移植肾功能延迟恢复	2.7
急性排斥反应	10.1
感染	20.1
移植受者死亡	4.0
移植肾全因丢失	5.4

4. 肾脏移植受者、移植物生存分析

2015 年至 2019 年期间全国范围内开展的肾脏移植共计 52,005 例，

进行移植受者 / 移植物（以下简称：人 / 肾）的生存分析，结果如下：

（1）移植术后 1 年生存率：DD 肾脏移植的 1 年人 / 肾生存率为 97.8% / 95.7%；亲属间活体肾脏移植的 1 年人 / 肾生存率为 99.4% / 98.8%（表 3-10）。

（2）移植术后 3 年生存率：DD 肾脏移植的 3 年人 / 肾生存率为 96.9% / 93.3%；亲属间活体肾脏移植的 3 年人 / 肾生存率为 98.9% / 97.0%（表 3-10）。

表 3-10　中国肾脏移植术后生存率（不包含港澳台地区）

供体类别	术后 1 年		术后 3 年	
	移植受者（%）	移植物（%）	移植受者（%）	移植物（%）
DD 肾脏	97.8	95.7	96.9	93.3
亲属间活体肾脏	99.4	98.8	98.9	97.0

四、特点与展望

1. DD 肾脏移植是当今主要的移植类型

自 2015 年起，公民逝世后器官捐献在我国得到了大力推动，2019 年 DD 肾脏移植占比 85.7%，以广东、湖北、山东、浙江、湖南等省份位居前列，区域优势较明显。近年来儿童肾脏移植以广东、河南、上海等省份开展较多。此外，2019 年儿童肾脏捐献者占比 7.7%。

器官的区域分配原则以及器官转运绿色通道的建立，缩短了 DD 肾脏移植的供肾冷缺血时间。亲属间活体肾脏移植和 DD 肾脏移植的 1 年、3 年移植肾生存率满意。2019 年肾脏相关的多器官联合移植 224 例，其中 66.5% 为胰肾联合移植，主要在天津、广东、湖南、广西和山东开展较多。

2. 持续开展肾脏移植质量控制与质量提升工程

质控中心宗旨是以建设符合中国肾脏移植学科发展特点的 CSRKT 为基石，发挥行业引领作用，加强人体器官移植医疗质量的管理，实现全国肾脏移植医疗质量和服务水平的持续改进，缩小各移植中心的医疗差距，一系列质控标准与技术规范由此出台。此外还根据这些技术规范制订了肾脏移植质量提升工程，进行前瞻性研究，从而实现从医学质量评价（控制）到医疗质量提升的良性循环，不断推进我国肾脏移植事业的发展。

3. 关注肾脏移植研究热点并取得突破性进展

在未来很长时间内，器官移植供体短缺和移植排斥反应依然是制约肾脏移植发展的关键因素。多年来，国内学者致力于将免疫学、干细胞和基因工程等领域的成果与器官移植紧密联系起来，大力开展基础与临床研究，为进一步优化肾脏移植医疗质量提供了理论和实践依据。在供者特异性抗体、抗体介导排斥反应、临床免疫耐受、潜在器官捐献者的器官功能维护、供体器官保存和充分利用、移植相关病毒感染等研究热点方面，已取得突破性进展。

4. 向国际器官移植界传递"中国之音"

CSRKT 是我国器官移植信息化建设的宝贵财富。肾脏移植质控中心在加强 CSRKT 科学性建设的同时进行数据挖掘，开展了大样本的中国肾脏移植受者临床结局的真实世界研究。研究报告在欧洲器官移植大会展示并在国际期刊 *Transplant International* 上发表，真实揭示了中国内地肾脏移植的特点、成绩、不足与展望。杂志社对此发表评论，指出"需要为中国移植中心的出色成绩而喝彩"。此外，质控中心还向 *World Medical Journal*、*Chinese Medical Journal* 杂志撰文，实事求是地论述了中国器官移植体系建设在探索中规范、在规范中成长的发展经验，向世界医学同道传递"中国之音"，用中国器官移植发展的事实有力驳斥某些别有用心的组织将移植政治化的相关谬论，表明中国器官移植工作者将不断加强自身建设，以符合伦理和世界卫生组织准则的方式发展中国器官移植事业。

第四章　中国心脏移植

本章内容主要基于中国心脏移植注册系统（China Heart Transplant Registry，CHTR）数据分析。数据统计范围是中国内地数据，不包含港澳台地区。

CHTR 是在国家卫生健康委督导下建立的、具有官方性质的心脏移植注册系统，要求全国具有心脏移植资质的医疗机构必须及时、完整地向其填报移植相关信息。CHTR 主要数据内容包括：受者基本情况、心脏供者情况、移植术中情况、免疫抑制剂应用情况、移植近期和远期结果。CHTR 通过对中国内地的心脏移植情况进行动态、科学地分析，定期发布各心脏移植中心手术量、数据质量和临床质量，并基于移植数据，发布心脏供体获取和保存、组织配型和移植围术期管理等方面的结果和经验，为国家监管部门制定移植相关的政策、法规提供科学依据。

一、心脏移植医疗机构分布

截至 2019 年 12 月 31 日，中国共有 57 所医疗机构具备心脏移植资质，与 2018 年相比增加 11 所。其中，心脏移植机构数量较多的省（区、市）为广东（6），浙江（6），北京（5）和湖北（5）（图 4-1）。

CHTR 数据显示，2015 年至 2019 年全国上报心脏移植手术共 2,262 例（图 4-2）。2019 年共有 38 家心脏移植医疗机构实施并上报心脏移植手术 679 例，移植例数比 2018 年增加了 38.6%，其中儿童（＜ 18 岁）心脏移植 59 例，心肺联合移植 8 例。各省（区、市）心脏移植例数分布如图 4-3 所示。2019 年，除港澳台地区外，中国心脏移植例数排名前十位的医疗机构见图4-4。

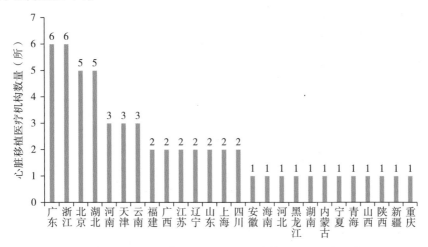

图 4-1　2019 年中国具有心脏移植医疗机构分布情况（不包含港澳台地区）

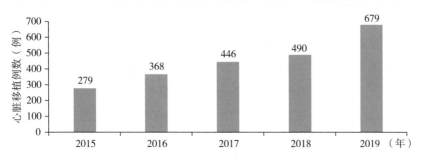

图 4-2　2015—2019 年中国心脏移植例数（不包含港澳台地区）

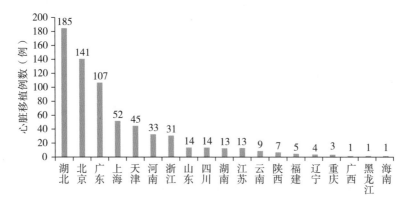

图 4-3　2019 年中国各省（区、市）心脏移植例数分布（不包含港澳台地区）

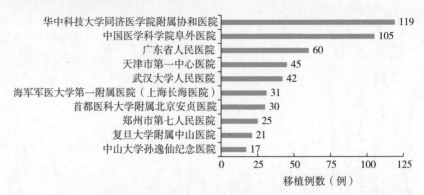

图 4-4　2019 年中国心脏移植例数排名前十位的医疗机构（不包含港澳台地区）

二、心脏移植受者人口特征

2019 年，心脏移植受者年龄中位数为 50.0 岁，其中，男性受者比例为 74.7%；受者 BMI 中位数为 22.3。移植受者血型中 O 型占 30.8%，A 型占 30.5%，B 型占 28.3%，AB 型占 10.4%。儿童移植受者年龄中位数为 11.0 岁，男性占比 49.1%（表 4-1）。心脏移植受者病因以非缺血性心肌病和冠心病为主，占比分别为 71.0% 和 13.7%，其余为先天性心脏病（4.3%），心脏瓣膜病（5.7%）以及其他病因（5.3%）。儿童受者病因以非缺血性心肌病（76.4%）和先天性心脏病（14.6%）为主。

表 4-1　2019 年中国心脏移植受者人口特征（不包含港澳台地区）

变量	总体移植受者	儿童移植受者
年龄中位数，IQR（岁）	50.0（35.0 ~ 57.0）	11.0（7.0 ~ 14.0）
男性占比（%）	74.7	49.1
体重中位数，IQR（kg）	62.5（52.0 ~ 71.0）	35.0（23.0 ~ 46.0）
身高中位数，IQR（cm）	168.0（162.0 ~ 173.0）	150.0（122.0 ~ 164.0）
BMI 中位数，IQR（kg/m²）	22.2（19.4 ~ 24.5）	16.1（13.9 ~ 18.9）
心脏移植病因占比（%）		
非缺血性心肌病	71.0	76.4
冠心病	13.7	0
先天性心脏病	4.3	14.6
心脏瓣膜病	5.7	3.6
其他疾病	5.3	5.4

注：IQR，interquartile range，四分位间距。

三、心脏移植质量安全分析

1. 心脏缺血时间

2019 年，全国心脏移植的缺血时间分布情况如图 4-5 所示。2019 年全国心脏移植心脏缺血时间中位数为 4.0 小时。心脏移植缺血时间大于 6 小时的移植受者占比为 15.6%，低于 2015—2018 年的 22.1%。

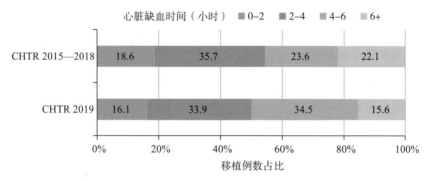

图 4-5　2019 年中国心脏移植心脏缺血时间情况（不包含港澳台地区）

2. 术后院内生存情况

2019 年，全国心脏移植受者院内存活率为 93.2%，其中，移植病因为心肌病和冠心病的受者院内存活率分别为 94.3% 和 91.4%。心脏移植受者术后感染发生率为 22.0%，其他术后主要并发症分别为心搏骤停（3.5%）、二次开胸（5.3%）、气管切开（4.7%）和二次插管（6.0%）。在心脏移植受者院内死亡原因情况中，多器官衰竭和移植心脏衰竭共占早期死亡原因的 50% 以上（表 4-2）。

表 4-2　2019 年心脏移植受者术后院内生存情况

变量	率 / 构成比（%）
院内存活	93.2
术后并发症	
院内感染	22.0
心搏骤停	3.5
二次开胸	5.3

续表

变量	率／构成比（%）
气管切开	4.7
二次插管	6.0
院内死亡原因	
多器官衰竭	39.6
移植心脏衰竭	12.5
感染	16.7
其他	31.3

3. 生存分析

2015 至 2019 年，全国心脏移植术后 1 年的生存率为 85.2%，3 年的术后生存率为 80.0%。其中，成人心脏移植术后的 1 年生存率和 3 年生存率分别为 84.7% 和 79.4%；儿童心脏移植术后的 1 年生存率和 3 年生存率分别为 92.6% 和 90.6%（表 4-3）。

表 4-3　2015—2019 年心脏移植术后生存率

	术后 1 年生存率（%）	术后 3 年生存率（%）
总体	85.2	80.0
成人	84.7	79.4
儿童	92.6	90.6

四、特点与展望

2019 年全国心脏移植例数增长较快，比 2018 年增加了 38.6%。2019 年增加了 11 家具备心脏移植资质的医疗机构，表明我国心脏移植的地区可及性在逐渐提升。2019 年，华中科技大学附属协和医院、中国医学科学院阜外医院和广东省人民医院 3 家心脏移植中心的年移植例数在 60 例以上，表明我国有 3 家心脏移植中心已进入国际心脏移植大中心的行列。

在心脏移植例数快速增长的情况下，2019 年我国心脏移植受者院内存活率和远期存活率均能保持稳中有升的趋势；在心脏供体缺血时间方面，得益于中国人体器官分配与共享计算机系统的高效运行以及各家移植医疗团队的不懈努力，心脏缺血时间在 6 小时以上的例数占比大幅度下降，以上显示了我国在心脏供体选择维护、受者围术期管理及术后长期管理方面已经积累了成功经验。

2019 年，国家心脏移植质控中心组织专家委员会，修订并发布了2019 年《中国心脏移植诊疗技术规范》《规范》涵盖心脏移植受者术前评估与准备，心脏移植供心获取与保护，心脏移植术操作规范、心脏移植免疫抑制治疗及排斥反应诊疗、术后并发症诊疗规范以及术后随访技术等章节内容。同时，通过学术讲座和资质进修培训，在全国范围内开展技术规范的讲解与培训，进一步加快了全国心脏移植相关技术的同质化进程。

展望未来，中国心脏移植质控中心将进一步完善中国心脏移植注册登记系统，建立与国际接轨的合作交流机制；通过专家委员会，制定心脏移植相关的质控标准体系和技术规范，同时督促技术规范的执行，加强心脏移植相关的技术培训，扶持技术和管理较弱的移植中心，逐步缩减地区差异。

第五章　中国肺脏移植

本章内容主要基于中国肺脏移植注册系统（China Lung Transplantation Registry, CLuTR）中的数据分析。数据范围为中国内地，不包含港澳台地区。

CLuTR 是中国目前唯一一个国家级的肺脏移植受者数据科学登记系统，全面及时地收集了受者术前、捐献者、受者手术、术后及随访信息。通过对中国内地的肺脏移植情况进行动态、科学地分析，为国家监管部门制定移植相关政策、法规提供依据。

一、肺脏移植医疗机构分布

2015 年至 2019 年，除港澳台地区外，我国共有 43 所医疗机构取得肺脏移植资质，覆盖全国 21 个省份，地理分布范围主要集中在东部和华北地区，其中河北、山西、吉林、江西、重庆、贵州、西藏、甘肃、青海和宁夏地区尚无医疗机构取得肺脏移植资质（图 5-1）。

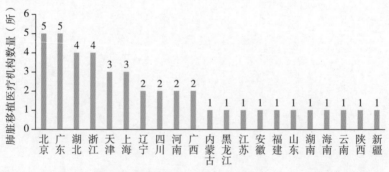

图 5-1　2019 年中国具有肺脏移植资质的医疗机构分布（不包含港澳台地区）

2015 年 1 月 1 日至 2019 年 12 月 31 日，CLuTR 共上报肺脏移植手术
1,513 例，各年度开展肺脏移植手术分别为 118、204、299、403 和 489 例（图
5-2），呈逐年上升趋势。

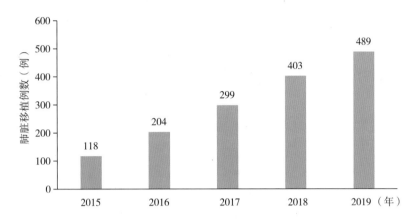

图 5-2　2015—2019 年中国肺脏移植手术数量（不包含港澳台地区）

2019 年，有 23 个中心开展了肺脏移植手术。手术数量居前三位的中
心分别为无锡市人民医院、中日友好医院和广州医科大学附属第一医院，
分别占总例数的 30.5%、20.0% 和 16.1%（图 5-3）。

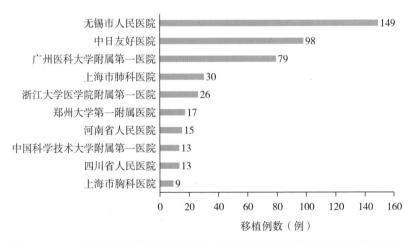

图 5-3　2019 年度中国肺脏移植例数前十位的医疗机构（不包含港澳台地区）

二、肺脏移植受者人口特征

2019 年我国肺脏移植单、双肺冷缺血时间中位数（IQR）分别为 6.0（4.0 ~ 7.0）h 和 8.0（6.2 ~ 9.3）h。单肺冷缺血时间＜2h、2 ~ 4h、4 ~ 6h、6 ~ 8h 及 ≥ 8h 的比例分别为 4.3%、27.5%、24.9%、37.7% 和 5.6%；双肺冷缺血时间相应比例分别为 2.2%、6.6%、15.8%、30.1% 和 45.3%（图 5-4）。

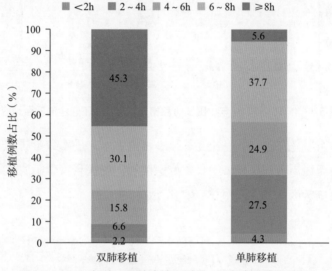

图 5-4　2019 年单、双肺冷缺血时间（不包含港澳台地区）

2019 年我国肺脏移植受者男性占 82.2%；年龄为（54.9 ± 12.8）岁，60 岁以上占 49.0%。BMI 为（20.3 ± 3.9）Kg/m^2；O、A、B 及 AB 血型分别占比 29.6%、32.3%、30.2% 及 7.9%。移植前 29.6% 的受者使用过激素药物，9.4% 的受者在 ICU 住院，日常活动完全受限（NYHA IV）以及病情严重需住院治疗的比例分别为 15.6% 和 12.5%（表 5-1）。

2019 年我国肺脏移植受者原发病中以特发性间质性肺炎、慢性阻塞性肺疾病及继发性间质性肺炎和尘肺为主，分别占 37.0%、20.9%、11.0% 和 10.2%。此外，支气管扩张症、肺动脉高压、闭塞性细支气管炎、移植

肺功能衰竭和淋巴管平滑肌瘤病分别占 7.8%、3.1%、2.2%、1.2% 和 1.0%
（图 5-5）。

表 5-1 2019 年肺脏移植受者人口特征（不包含港澳台地区）

变量	占比 (%)
性别	
男	82.2
女	17.8
年龄 (岁)	
＜ 18	1.8
18 ~ 35	10.0
36 ~ 49	15.7
50 ~ 59	23.5
60 ~ 64	27.7
≥ 65	21.3
BMI 分级（Kg/m^2）	
＜ 18.5	33.5
18.6 ~ 23.9	46.0
≥ 24.0	20.5
血型	
O 型	29.6
A 型	32.3
B 型	30.2
AB 型	7.9
激素药物治疗史	
有	29.6
无	70.4
移植前住院情况	
ICU	9.4
普通住院	75.1
未住院	15.5
移植前心功能状态	
无活动限制（NYHA I/II）	1.4
日常活动部分受限（NYHA III）	70.5
日常活动完全受限（NYHA IV）	15.6
病情严重需住院治疗	12.5

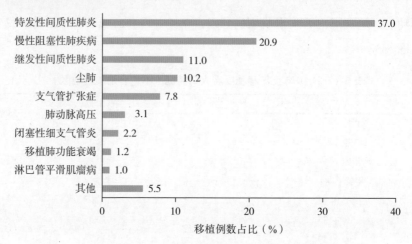

图 5-5　2019 年我国肺脏移植受者原发病分布 (不包含港澳台地区)

三、肺脏移植质量安全分析

1. 手术方式

2019 年我国肺脏移植术中单、双肺移植分别占 45.0% 和 55.0%。急诊肺移植占 14.0%，术中使用体外膜肺氧合（Extracorporeal Membrane Oxygenation，ECMO）的比例为 60.2%。

2. 术中输血

术中输血量的中位数(IQR)为 1,065.0(600.0 ~ 1,790.0)mL，< 500mL、500 ~ 999mL、1,000 ~ 1,499mL、1,500 ~ 1,999mL 和 ≥ 2,000mL 的比例分别为 18.6%、23.7%、21.1%、15.1% 和 21.5%。

3. 术后早期（< 30 天）并发症

术后早期并发症主要包括感染（65.2%）、肾功能不全（30.9%）、原发性肺移植物失功（18.3%）、糖尿病（15.9%）、急性排斥反应（8.4%）和气管吻合口病变（6.4%）（图 5-6）。

4. 出院时状态

2019 年我国肺脏移植受者住院时间中位数(IQR)为 30.0(19.0 ~ 49.0)天，出院前存活率为 75.8%。受者围术期死因主要为肺部感染导致的休克或呼吸循环衰竭（27.7%）、多器官功能衰竭（27.7%）、原发性肺移植物失功（13.8%）和心源性猝死（10.8%）（图5-7）。

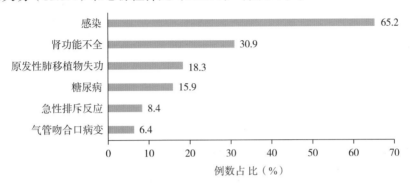

图5-6　2019年我国肺脏移植受者围术期并发症（不包含港澳台地区）

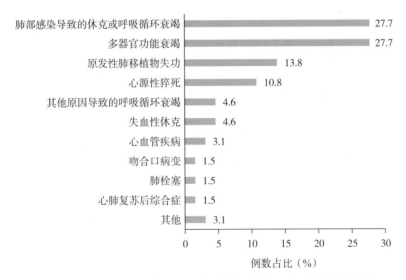

图5-7　2019年我国肺脏移植受者围术期死因（不包含港澳台地区）

5. 术后生存状况

我国双肺移植受者术后围手术期（＜30天）、3个月、6个月、1年及3年生存率分别为78.8%、69.3%、65.3%、63.5%和56.1%，单肺移植受者相应生存率分别为84.2%、77.7%、73.5%、68.7%和52.3%，单肺移植受者近期生存率优于双肺移植受者（表5-2）。

表 5-2　中国肺脏移植术后受者生存率（不包含港澳台地区）

项目	围手术期（＜30天）	3个月	6个月	1年	3年
双肺（%）	78.8	69.3	65.3	63.5	56.1
单肺（%）	84.2	77.7	73.5	68.7	52.3

四、特点与展望

近年来，国家肺脏移植质控中心不断完善肺移植临床诊疗体系，推广规范化肺移植技术。2019 年我国肺移植例数相比 2018 年增长迅速，继续保持了全国肺移植数量上升势头。2019 年，在儿童肺移植领域取得了较大进步和突破，但急诊肺移植、术后感染、原发性移植物失功、心源性猝死、肾功能不全等术后并发症发生率仍然较高。

1. 国内首届国际肺脏移植论坛成功举办，推动中国肺移植早日进入世界移植舞台的中央

2019 年 11 月 2 日，国内首届国际肺移植论坛在无锡成功举办。论坛吸引了来自美国克利夫兰医学中心、意大利米兰大学医学院、日本东京大学医学院、韩国首尔峨山医学中心和蔚山医学院等多国专家教授，以及香港玛丽医院、台湾林口长庚医院等胸心外科专家出席。会议围绕肺移植学科的内外科技术、麻醉、护理及基础研究等方面的经验和新进展进行交流，开展了病例交流和讨论等形式多样、内容丰富的学术活动。此次论坛为国内外心肺移植专家提供了高水平的交流机会，有助于推动中国移植事业不断发展。未来，中国的肺移植事业将进一步与国际接轨，更好地融入国际移植学界的大家庭，为全人类的医学发展做出更大贡献。

2. 继续提升儿童肺移植临床技术

目前儿童肺移植仍然是国内肺移植的瓶颈，2015 年至 2018 年期间，全国共完成 8 例年龄 18 岁以下的儿童肺移植，围术期生存率均欠佳。但2019 年全国共完成 9 例儿童肺移植，创下了国内年龄最小的儿童肺移植记录和年度开展儿童肺移植例数最多的记录，目前儿童受者整体状态良

好。鉴于儿童在身体机能、生长发育、免疫排异等方面均与成人存在较大不同，儿童肺移植临床管理仍存在不少技术难关有待进一步攻克。

3. 贯彻落实肺移植术前评估制度，减少急诊肺移植

相比 2015 年至 2018 年，2019 年肺移植受者的术前心功能状态和 ICU 住院比例均更低，但急诊肺移植比例却更高。急诊肺移植患者病情危重、时间仓促，移植存在更大风险，术后发生排斥反应及原发性移植物失功的危险较高，术后围手术期生存率及近远期生存率也更低。因此，应进一步推动肺移植术前评估制度，严格把关受者的移植禁忌证和适应证。

4. 加大术后并发症监测和控制力度

2019 年肺移植术后感染发生率和前几年相当，但原发性移植物失功、心源性猝死、肾功能不全等并发症发生率却显著上升。对感染控制，应建立全程化、多环节的感控机制，从术前评估、供者质量维护、手术操作和术后管理多个层面做好感染预防和控制工作。对原发性移植物失功的防治，应充分把好供体质量关，对身体机能较差的受者可考虑使用体外循环辅助技术或适当延长 ECMO 转流时间。对心源性猝死的防治，要重视术前受者心功能状态的评估，术后要动态监测心功能状态，对心功能异常者，要予以积极处理。对肾功能不全的防治，要重视药物浓度和肾功能指标的监测，尤其要注意药物之间的相互作用，尽量避免加重肾脏负担。

尽管我国肺移植近年来发展迅速，但与国际心肺移植协会报道的生存率相比，仍存在一定差距。主要原因在于与国际肺移植情况相比，我国肺移植受者年龄大、病情危重、手术难度大、肺纤维化患者多，且公民逝世后捐献供肺的呼吸机使用时间长、冷缺血时间长。后期，肺移植质控中心将进一步修订肺脏移植技术临床应用质量控制指标，完善肺移植标准流程和技术规范，持续打造多学科联合的肺移植团队，构建完备的肺移植数据库、挖掘数据资源，继续提升肺移植质量。

Chapter 1   Human Organ Allocation and Sharing in China

This chapter was generated based on the data of the China Organ Transplant Response System (COTRS). The data scope of statistics was from Mainland China date of HongKong, Macao, and Taiwan was not included.

From January 1st, 2015 to December 31st, 2019, there were 24,112 donors of deceased donations (DDs) in total. In 2019, 5,818 DD donors recorded, and 19,454 patients received organ transplantation in China. The rate of donation rose from 2.01 pmp (donors permillion population) in 2015 to 4.16 pmp in 2019.

China organ donation and transplant scheme (Figure 1-1) is consists of the organ donation system, organ procurement and allocation system, organ transplant service system, quality control system, regulatory system, to achieve an open, fair and transparent organ allocation.

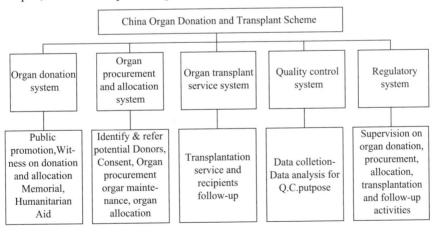

Figure 1-1   China organ donation and transplant scheme
(Hongkong, Macao and Taiwan not included)

COTRS an essential part of China organ donation and transplant Scheme and is composed of three subsystems—the "potential organ donor identification system", "organ donor registration and organ matching system", and "organ transplantation waiting list system" and the supervision platform.

The COTRS is a manifestation of laws on organ transplantation and donation in articles 6 and 22 in the "Regulations on Human Organ Transplantation" and article 234 of the "Amendment VIII to the Criminal Law". In 2018, the National Health Commission issued the "Notice on Issuing the Basic Principles and Core Policies for China Organ Allocation and Sharing" (GWYF〔2018〕No. 24) revising the "Notice of the Ministry of Health on Issuing the Basic Principles for China Organ Allocation and Sharing and the Core Policies for Liver and Kidney Transplantation" (WYGF〔2010〕No. 113); developed the core policies for heart and lung allocation and sharing; and formulated the "Basic Principles and Core Policies for China Organ Allocation and Sharing".

COTRS implements the national scientific organ allocation policy by automatically allocating and sharing organs and providing full monitoring for national and local regulators so as to establish the traceability of organ procurement and allocation, minimize human intervention and ensure a just, fair, and open allocation of organs. Moreover, it functions as an essential cornerstone for winning people's trust in the work of DD.

COTRS, certified by the China Information Technology Security Evaluation Center, guarantees the information security of donors and recipients during the organ allocation and protects patient privacy by controlling the access and monitoring the operations of relevant medical institutions. It consists of three subsystems, i.e., Potential Organ Donor Identification & referral System, Organ Donor Registry and Organ Matching System, Organ Transplant Waiting List System, with a supervision platform.

1.1 Distribution of medical institations for organ donation and transplantation

1.1.1 Distribution of OPO in China

In China organ donation and transplant scheme, the OPO, set up in a medical institution, is composed of medical personnel, organ donation coordinators and administrative staff. which is different from that of the United States and Spain's Organization National De Transplantz (ONT).

By December 31st, 2019, China had 125 OPOs (Figure 1-2).

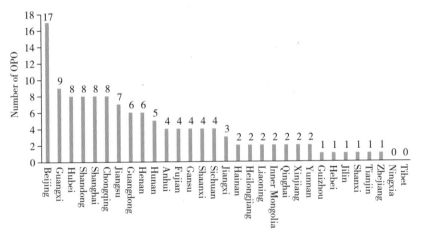

Figure 1-2   Distribution of OPO by province of China in 2019

(Hongkong, Macao and Taiwan not included)

1.1.2 Distribution of transplant centers in China

By December 31st, 2019, there were 173 medical institutions qualified for organ transplantation in China (Figure 1-3), and the top 5 provinces were Guangdong (19), Beijing (17), Shandong (13), Shanghai (11), Hunan (9) and Zhejiang (9).

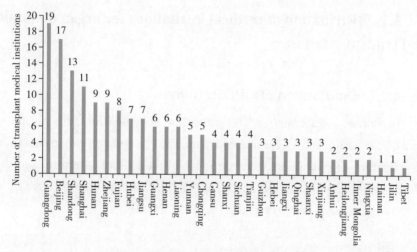

Figure 1-3   Distribution of transplantation medical institutions of China in 2019
(Hongkong, Macao and Taiwan not included)

1.2   Organ donation

1.2.1   Organ donation in China

During 2015–2019, the number of DD was 2,766; 4,080; 5,146; 6,302; and 5,818, and the PMP was 2.01, 2.98, 3.72, 4.53 and 4.16 (Figure 1-4).

During 2015–2019, the top 5 provinces of China based on the number of organ donations were Guangdong (3,290), Hubei (2,472), Shandong (2,428), Hunan (2,126), and Beijing (1,898) (Figure 1-5).

In 2019, the top 5 provinces of China based on the number of organ donations were Guangdong (890), Hubei (599), Shandong (495), Tianjin (457), and Hunan (429). Qinghai achieved at least one human organ donation.

The PMP exceeded the national level in 12 provinces (4.16). The top 5 provinces were Tianjin (29.29), Beijing (13.79), Hubei (10.12), Guangdong (7.84), and Hainan (7.60). Figure 1-6 shows the PMPs of the provinces in 2019.

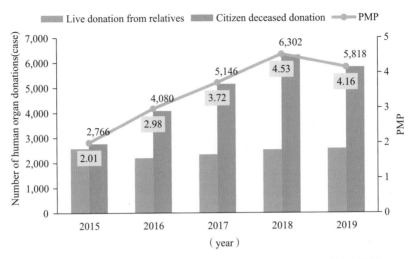

Figure 1-4 Number of Organ Donations of China during 2015–2019

(Hongkong, Macao and Taiwan not included)

Note: The population in 2015–2017 was obtained from the *China Health Statistics Yearbook.*

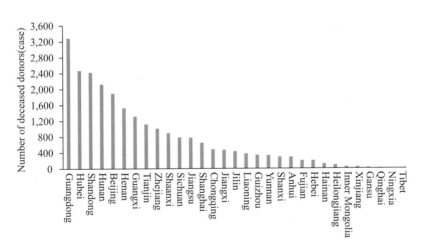

Figure 1-5 Number of DD by provinces during 2015–2019

(Hongkong, Macao and Taiwan not included)

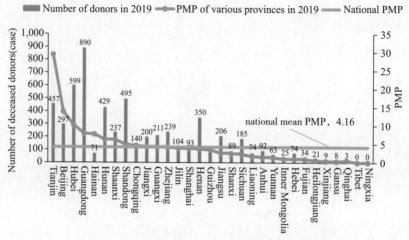

Figure 1-6   Number of DD and PMP by province in 2019
(Hongkong, Macao and Taiwan not included)

During the 5-year period from 2015 to 2019, 10 OPOs performed more than 600 DDs, 10 OPOs performed 300-600 DDs, 15 OPOs performed 200-299 DDs. In 2019, 3 OPOs performed more than 200 DDs, 10 OPOs wore between 100-200 DDs and 23 OPOs wore between 50-99 DDs.

1.2.2 Characteristics of deceased donors

In 2019, the median age of the deceased donors was 47, and child donors (under the age of 18) accounted for 8.20%. 81.57% of the donors were males. Per the blood type, 38.12% of the donors were blood Type O, 28.45% were blood Type A, 25.95% were blood Type B, and 7.48% were blood Type AB (Figure 1-7). Notably, 32.76% of the donations were C-I (donation after brain death, DBD), 44.35% were C-II (donation after cardiac death, DCD), and 22.89% were C-III (donation after brain death followed by cardiac death, DBCD) (Figure 1-8).

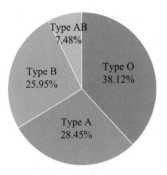

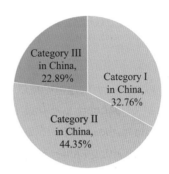

Figure 1-7   Blood type deceased donors (Hongkong, Macao and Taiwan not included)

Figure 1-8   Category of deceased donors (Hongkong, Macao and Taiwan not included)

During 2015–2019, trauma and cerebrovascular accidents were the two main causes of deceased donors' death, accounting for 86.82% of all death (Figure 1-9). The proportion of donors who died due to cerebrovascular accidents increased year by year. In 2019, cerebrovascular accidents overtook trauma as the leading cause of death in Chinese deceased organ donors (Figure 1-10).

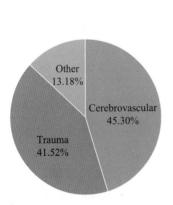

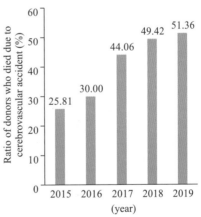

Figure 1-9   Causes of deceased donors' death (Hongkong, Macao and Taiwan not included)

Figure 1-10   Proportion of donors with cerebro-vascular accident in 2015–2019 (Hongkong, Macao and Taiwan not included)

1.3   Patients waiting for organ transplantation

During 2015–2019, the number of patients waiting for liver and kidney transplantation (Figure 1-11) increased by year. During 2017–2019, the number of patients awaiting liver transplantation annually was significantly higher than those in 2015 and 2016. By the end of 2019, there were 47,382 patients awaiting kidney and 4,763 patients awaiting liver. The heart and lung allocation system began its operation on October 22, 2018. By the end of 2019, 338 and 89 people were still awaiting heart and lung transplantation, respectively.

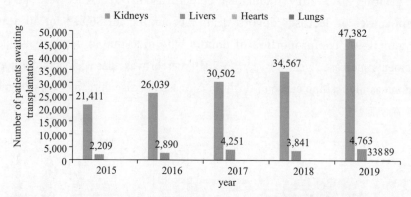

Figure 1-11   Number of patients awaiting organ transplantation during 2015–2019 (Hongkong, Macao and Taiwan not included)

Figure 1-12 shows the top 5 provinces based on the number of patients waiting for kidney transplantation were Guangdong (6,105), Zhejiang (5,155), Hunan (4,937), Sichuan (3,724), and Shanghai (3,644), at the end of 2019.

Figure 1-13 shows the top 5 provinces based on the number of patients waiting for liver transplantation were Sichuan (1,142), Guangdong (805), Tianjin (558), Shanghai (372), and Beijing (298), at the end of 2019.

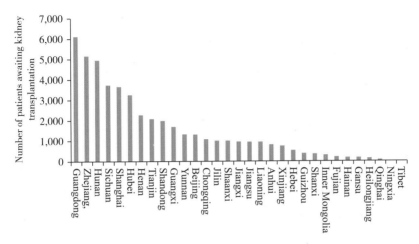

Figure 1-12   Number of patients awaiting kidney transplantation at the end of 2019 by province (Hongkong, Macao and Taiwan not included)

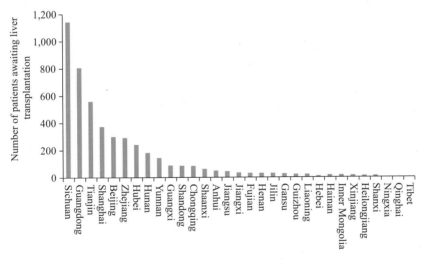

Figure 1-13   Number of patients awaiting liver transplantation at the end of 2019 by province (Hongkong, Macao and Taiwan not included)

Figure 1-14 shows the top 5 provinces based on the number of patients waiting for heart transplantation were Beijing (108), Guangdong (37), Hubei (30), Shanghai (25), and Zhejiang (23), at the end of 2019.

53

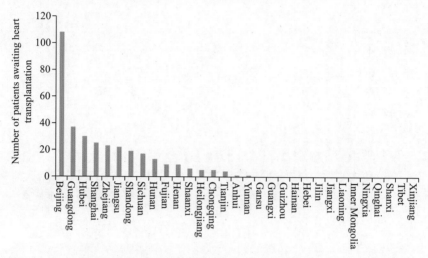

Figure 1-14   Number of patients awaiting heart transplantation at the end of 2019 by province (Hongkong, Macao and Taiwan not included)

Figure 1-15 shows the top 5 provinces based on the number of patients waiting for lung transplantation were Guangdong (21), Jiangsu (13), Hubei (12), Shanghai (10), and Zhejiang (9), at the end of 2019.

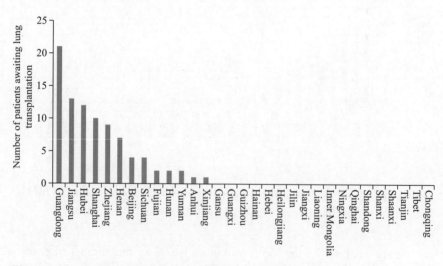

Figure 1-15   Number of patients awaiting lung transplantation at the end of 2019 by province (Hongkong, Macao and Taiwan not included)

1.4　Utilization of organs

1.4.1　The yield of donated organs per donor

During 2015–2019, the yield of donated kidney organs per donor by year was 1.92, 1.87, 1.89, 1.91, and 1.89, and that of liver was 0.88, 0.87, 0.90, 0.91, and 0.93 (Figure 1-16). In 2019, the mean number of hearts harvested from each donor was 0.12, and the mean number of lungs harvested from each donor was 0.15.

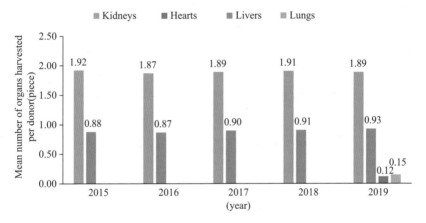

Figure 1-16　The yield of donated organs per donor in 2015–2019

(Hongkong, Macao and Taiwan not included)

1.4.2　Comparison of organ sharing before and after the imple–mentation of the green channel policy

On May 6th, 2016, the then National Health and Family Planning Commission, the Ministry of Public Security, the Ministry of Transportation, the Civil Aviation Administration of China, China Railway, and the Red Cross Society of China jointly issued the "Notice on Establishing a Green channel for organ Transportation" (here in after referred to as the "Notice") to establish a green channel for donated organ transportation. In the "Notice", responsibilities of all parties were specified, aiming to ensure smooth transportation of organs and minimize the impact of organ transportation time on the quality and safety of organ transplant patients.

In the "Notice", organ transportation was divided into general and emergency processes based on the transportation type to achieve a fast track and priority transportation of organs, to improve the efficiency and guarantee the safety of the transportation, and to reduce the organ wastage owing to transportation.

Comparison of organ sharing in China before and after the implementation of the green channel policy for organ transportation reveals that after the implementation of the policy, the sharing of livers and kidneys (Table 1-1) in China has increased by 7.8%, of which the sharing of kidneys increased by 5.9%, and the sharing of livers increased by 6.4%.

Table 1-1 Sharing of livers and kidney in China before and after the implementation of the Green Channel Policy (%) (excluding Hong Kong, Macau, and Taiwan)

Period	Overall (%)			Kidney (%)			Liver (%)		
	Before	After	Change	Before	After	Change	Before	After	Change
For center level use	75.0	66.5	−8.5	84.6	77.6	−7.0	53.2	48.7	−4.5
Shared within the province	12.6	13.3	0.7▲	10.5	11.6	1.1▲	17.3	15.4	−1.9
National sharing	12.4	20.2	7.8▲	4.9	10.8	5.9▲	29.5	35.9	6.4▲

1.5 Summary and prospects

Organ transplantation is a significant achievement in the development of human medicine, and it has saved the lives of countless patients with end-stage diseases. In 2018, China ranked second worldwide, both in the number of DD and in the number of transplantalion.

1.5.1 Improving the utilization of donated organs

China has a large population and a large number of patients. Organ shortage is still one of the main factors in the development of organ transplantation. With the shortage of donated organs, it is necessary to improve the maintenance of donated organs, expand the supply of organs, improve the utilization of heart and lung for transplantations, and increase the overall utilization of organs.

In addition, publicity and education on organ donation should be strengthened to raise public awareness.

1.5.2   Strengthening the role of green channel to reduce organ wastage during transportation

With the increase of organ donation in China, more and more organs are being matched and shared. The green channel policy for organ transportation helps to achieve a fast track and priority transportation of organs, to improve the efficiency and guarantee the safety of transportation, and to reduce the organ wastage owing to transportation.

1.5.3   Driving the conversion of high-speed growth and development to high-quality development in organ donation

Recently, the quantity and quality of organ donations and transplantations in China have been continuously increasing. With the improvements in medical conditions and increase in public expectations toward health, a huge gap remains between the public's needs for transplantation services and the uneven and insufficient development of the transplantation industry.

Promoting the conversion from high-speed growth and development to high-quality development in organ donation is important while focusing on the quantity and speed. While actively promoting organ donation, the clinical service resource layout for organ transplantation should be optimized; efforts should be made to solve the uneven development of organ transplantation techniques between regions and disciplines; and the level of donation, harvesting, and allocation management should be strengthened. Continuous growth in quantity should be maintained while increasing the quality, and efforts should be made to achieve a higher-quality, more efficient, fairer, and more sustainable development.

Chapter 2   Liver Transplantation in China

This chapter mainly analyzes the cases collected by the China Liver Transplant Registry (CLTR). These data are from Mainland China, excluding those from Hongkong, Macao and Taiwan.

CLTR is China's official liver transplant registry system established under the supervision of the National Health Commission, and it requires the medical institutions qualified to perform liver transplantation to report regarding the transplantation timely and entirely. CLTR describes the medical quality status of liver transplantation through the dynamic and scientific analysis of liver transplantation in Mainland China, provides a basis for national regulatory authorities to formulate relevant transplantation policies and regulations, and provides scientific management tools of liver transplant recipients to all transplant centers. Moreover, it has become one of the most significant information systems in organ transplantation and one of the academic exchange platforms for liver transplantation in China.

2.1   Distribution of medical institutions for liver transplantation

By December 31, 2019, there were 105 medical institutions qualified for liver transplantation in China, and they were mainly distributed in Beijing (12), Guangdong (12), Shanghai (9), Shandong (8), and Zhejiang (6) (Figure 2-1).

During 2015–2019, there were 23,890 liver transplantations in China, including 20,630 deceased donor liver transplantations (DDLTs) (86.4%) and 3,260 living donor liver transplantations (LDLTs) (13.6%). There were 19,760 adult liver transplants (82.7%) and 4,130 pediatric liver transplants (17.3%).

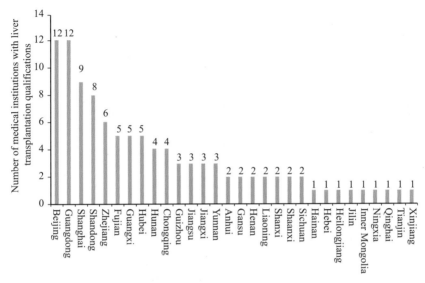

Figure 2-1   Distribution of medical institutions qualified for liver transplantation in China by the end of 2019 (Hongkong, Macao and Taiwan not included)

In 2019, there were 6,170 liver transplantations in China, including 5,332 DDLTs (86.4%) and 838 LDLTs (including 7 cases of domino liver transplantations) (13.6%). There were 5,075 adult liver transplantations (82.3%) and 1,095 pediatric liver transplantations (17.7%). In 2019, the top 5 provinces according to the number of liver transplantations were Shanghai (1,267), Guangdong (664), Beijing (605), Tianjin (602), and Zhejiang (586). In 2019, 14 provinces had 100 or more liver transplantations, accounting for 92.4% of the total number of liver transplantations in China (Figure 2-2). No liver transplantation was performed in Inner Mongolia and Ningxia in 2019. (There is no medical institution with liver transplantation qualification in Tibet at the present.)

In 2019, 10 medical institutions performed 200 or more liver transplantations, which accounted for 50.6% of all liver transplantations in China (Table 2-1).

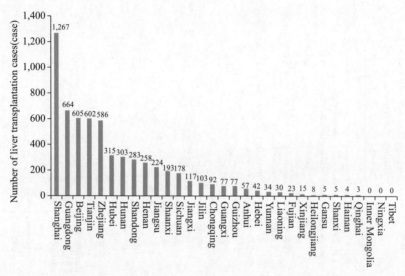

Figure 2-2   Distribution of liver transplantation in different provinces of China in 2019 (Hongkong, Macao and Taiwan not included)

Figure 2-1   Top 10 medical institutions according to the number of liver transplantations in 2019 (Hongkong, Macao and Taiwan not included)

Region	Liver transplantation medical institution	Number of patients
Shanghai	Renji Hospital Affiliated to Shanghai Jiaotong University School of Medicine	688
Tianjin	Tianjin First Central Hospital	602
Zhejiang	The First Affiliated Hospital of Zhejiang University	280
Guangdong	Third Affiliated Hospital, Sun Yat-Sen University	252
Shanghai	Zhongshan Hospital Affiliated to Fudan University	244
Shanghai	Huashan Hospital Affiliated to Fudan University	226
Zhejiang	Shulan (Hang Zhou) Hospital	221
Henan	First Affiliated Hospital of Zhengzhou University	208
Hunan	The Second Xiangya Hospital of Central South University	201
Beijing	Beijing Friendship Hospital, Capital Medical University	200

2.2   Data of liver transplant recipients

In 2019, the mean age of liver transplantation recipients in China was 42.2 years, and the median age was 48.7 years. The mean body mass index (BMI) of recipients was 22.3 kg/m^2, and the median BMI was 22.5 kg/m^2. Most recipients (75.0%) were male and had O, A, and B blood types with each accounting for approximately 30%, and recipients with blood type AB were the minority (Table 2-2).

Table 2-2   Demographic characteristics of Chinese liver transplant recipients in 2019 (Hongkong, Macao and Taiwan not included)

Variable	Mean ± standard deviation	Proportion (%)
Age (years)	42.2 ± 20.8	--
BMI(kg/m^2)	22.3 ± 4.4	--
Sex		
Male	--	75.0
Female	--	25.0
Blood type		
O	--	30.2
A	--	30.5
B	--	29.0
AB	--	10.3

2.3   Quality and safety analysis of liver transplantation

2.3.1   Important clinical markers for liver transplantation

In 2019, the mean cold ischemia time, mean anhepatic phase duration, mean intraoperative blood loss volume, and intraoperative mean red blood cell (RBC) transfusion volume for LDLTs were lower than those for DDLTs in China, and the mean duration of surgery for LDLTs was slightly higher than that for DDLTs (Figures 2.3-2.7).

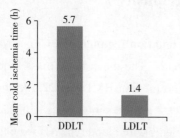

Figure 2-3　Mean cold ischemia time of DD liver transplantation in 2019 (Hongkong, Macao and Taiwan not included)

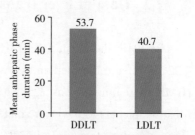

Figure 2-4　Mean anhepatic phase of DD liver transplantation in 2019 (Hongkong, Macao and Taiwan not included)

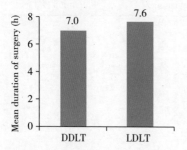

Figure 2-5　Mean operative time of DD liver transplantation in 2019 (Hongkong, Macao and Taiwan not included)

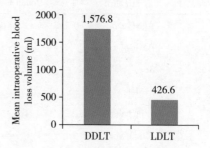

Figure 2-6　Mean blood loss during the operation of DD liver transplant-ation in 2019 (Hongkong, Macao and Taiwan not included)

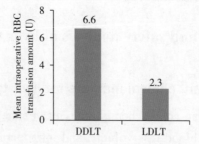

Figure 2-7　Mean volume of transfused RBC during the operation of DD liver transplantation in 2019 (Hongkong, Macao and Taiwan not included)

2.3.2　Changes in total bilirubin before and after liver transplantation in recipients

The changes in total bilirubin before and after liver transplantation in DDLT and LDLT recipients in 2019 were analyzed. The results showed that the mean total bilirubin significantly decreased after surgery (Table 2-3).

Table 2-3　Mean total bilirubin before and after liver transplantation in 2019 (Hongkong, Macao and Taiwan not included)

Time	Mean total bilirubin (μmol/L)	
	DDLT	LDLT
Before surgery	214.1	227.5
1 week after surgery	62.3	48.3
2 weeks after surgery	45.3	25.6
1 month after surgery	30.6	17.7
3 months after surgery	20.4	11.8
6 months after surgery	21.0	12.4

2.3.3　Condition of recipients after liver transplantation

(1) Complications within 30 days after surgery

In 2019, the incidence of complications within 30 days after surgery in DDLT recipients in China was 33.9%. Complications mainly included pleural effusion (19.7%), postoperative infection (15.4%), and ascites/abdominal abscess (12.9%). In addition, the incidence of complications within 30 days after surgery in LDLT recipients in China was 16.5%. Complications mainly included postoperative infection (8.1%), ascites/abdominal abscess (5.4%), and pleural effusion (3.7%).

(2) 30-day postoperative mortality rate

In 2019, the 30-day postoperative mortality rates for DDLT and LDLT recipients in China were 5.3% and 2.7%, respectively.

(3) Recipient and graft survival after liver transplantation

Survival analysis was performed for recipients and grafts for liver transplantation cases in China from 2015 to 2019.

The results were as follows: The postoperative 1-year and 3-year cumulative survival rates for DDLT recipients in China were 83.3% and 74.4%, respectively. Furthermore, the postoperative 1-year and 3-year cumulative survival rates for LDLT recipients in China were 91.8% and 88.5%, respectively.

The results are as follows: The postoperative 1-year and 3-year cumulative survival rates for DDLT grafts in China were 82.5% and 73.2%, respectively. The postoperative 1-year and 3-year cumulative survival rates for LDLT grafts in China were 91.3% and 87.5%, respectively (Table 2-4).

Table 2-4　Postoperative survival rate of liver transplantation recipients and grafts during 2015–2019 in China (Hongkong, Macao and Taiwan not included)

Group	Postoperative 1-year survival rate (%)		Postoperative 3-year survival rate (%)	
	Recipient	Graft	Recipient	Graft
DDLT	83.3	82.5	74.4	73.2
LDLT	91.8	91.3	88.5	87.5

(4) Tumor-free survival of recipients after liver transplantation

During 2015–2019, the postoperative 1-year and 3-year disease-free survival rates for patients with liver cancer who underwent liver transplantation were 77.6% and 62.5%, respectively.

2.4　Summary and prospects

Recently, the quantity and quality of liver transplantations in China have steadily increased to become at the top globally. In 2019, the number of liver transplantations in China was maintained at more than 6,000 cases.

2.4.1　Liver transplantation develops rapidly in pediatric

In 2019, the proportion of liver transplantation in pediatic was 17.7% in China. In China, Renji Hospital Affiliated to Shanghai Jiaotong University School of Medicine, which has the largest numher of pediatric liver transplantation, performed 443 cases of pediatric liver transplantations in 2019.

2.4.2 Most pediatric liver transplantation cases were LDLTs

In 2019, the proportion of living-related donor liver transplantation was 13.6% (n=838) in China. 70.4% of the liver allograft came from living-related donors among pediatric liver transplantation, which indicates a close relationship between relatives in China.

2.4.3 The proportion of liver transplantation for primary liver cancer was the highest among all liver transplantation cases

China has a high incidence of liver cancer. In 2019, 42.1% of DDLT recipients had malignancies. The Hangzhou criteria for liver transplantation of HCC has been widely recognized by the academic community and clinically applied. These criteria ensure that no significant difference in survival between China and other countries worldwide while simultaneously expanding the enrollment scope for patients with liver cancer to undergo liver transplantation.

2.4.4   Continuous search for innovation in surgical liver transplantation procedures and techniques

The anastomosis site has been changed from the gastroduodenal artery to the splenic artery, significantly improving the postoperative blood flow of the liver graft and reduces the incidence of biliary complications; a non-ischemic liver transplantation has been performed; the world's first auxiliary Domino liver transplantation has been performed by exchanging half of the liver of two individuals with different genetic metabolic defects to achieve organ transplantation without additional organ donation.

2.4.5   The standards and systems for quality management and control of liver transplantation need to be established and implemented.

The evaluation and preservation system of donated livers need to be further improved to improve the quality of donated livers, reduce the incidence of complications, and raise the survival rate of recipients. Furthermore, significant postoperative complications need to be extensively monitored, such as early allograft dysfunction, acute kidney injury, and new-onset diabetes. In addition,a more scientific and refined quality control system needs to be established to improve the clinical quality, service, and curative effect of liver transplantation in China.

2.4.6 Data on liver transplantation needs to be scientifically monitored to find valuable information.

Clinical research needs to be conducted using big data design and refined management, and clinical decisions have to be guided by evidence-based medicine. Therefore, superior clinical resources need to be gathered to innovate the multi-center, high-quality clinical research that focuses on the liver transplantation to facilitate the transformation from scientific findings to clinical application and promote the development of liver transplantation.

Chapter 3　Kidney Transplantation in China

This chapter is mainly based on the data from the Chinese Scientific Registry of Kidney Transplantation (CSRKT). Statistical limits are data from mainland of China, not including Hongkong, Macao and Taiwan.

CSRKT is China's official kidney transplant registry system established under the supervision of the National Health Commission, and it requires the medical institutions qualified to perform kidney transplantation to provide information regarding the transplantation timely and entirely. Being the unique scientific registry system of kidney transplant recipients in China, CSRKT provides bases for national regulatory authorities to formulate relevant transplantation policies and regulations through the dynamic and scientific analysis of kidney transplantation in China, and it provides scientific management tools of kidney transplant recipients to all transplant centers. Nowadays, it has become one of the most critical information systems in organ transplantation and academic exchange platforms for kidney transplantation in China.

3.1　Distribution of medical institutions for kidney transplantation

By December 31, 2019, there were total 135 medical institutions qualified for kidney transplantation in China, and they were mainly distributed in Guangdong (18), Beijing (13), Shandong (11), Hunan (9), and Zhejiang (8) (Figure 3-1).

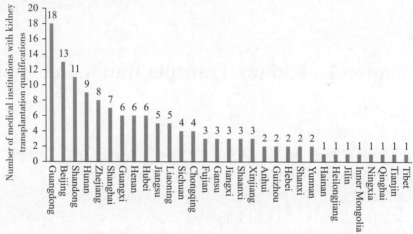

Figure 3-1 Geographical distribution of medical institutions qualifited for kidney transplantation in China (Hongkong, Macao and Taiwan not included)

During 2015–2019, overall 52,005 patients underwent kidney transplantation in China, of which 42,886 underwent DD kidney transplantation and 9,119 underwent living-related donor kidney transplantations. In 2019, 12,124 patients underwent kidney transplantations of which 10,389 underwent DD kidney transplantations, which was a decrease of 8.1% compared with that in 2018. There were 1,735 underwent living-related donor kidney transplantations, which was a decrease of 6.9% compared with that in 2018 (Figure 3-2).

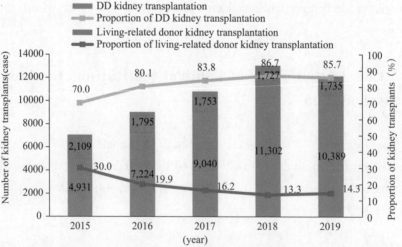

Figure 3-2 Number and proportion of DD kidney transplantations cases during 2015–2019 in China (Hongkong, Macao and Taiwan not included)

In 2019, 224 kidney-related multi-organ transplantations were performed in China. Among these transplantations, 68 were combined liver-kidney transplantations, 149 were combined pancreas-kidney transplantations, and 7 were combined heart-kidney transplantations. This was an increase of 45.5% compared with that in 2018 (Figure 3-3).

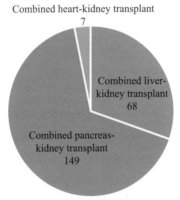

Figure 3-3　Number of kidney-related multi-organ transplantations in China in 2019 (Hongkong, Macao and Taiwan not included)

In 2019, the top 5 provinces based on the number of kidney-related multi-organ transplantations cases were Tianjin (69), Guangdong (66), Hunan (16), Guangxi (15), and Shandong (12) (Figure 3-4). Table 3-1 shows the top 10 medical institutions according to the number of kidney-related multi-organ transplantations in China.

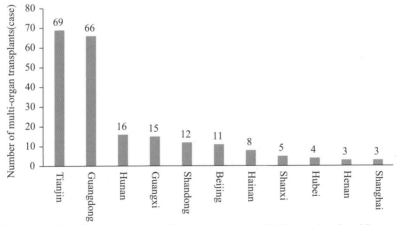

Figure 3-4　Top 10 provinces according to the number of kidney-related multi-organ transplantations in China in 2019 (Hongkong, Macao and Taiwan not included)

Table 3-1　Top 10 medical institutions according to the number of kidney-related multi-organ transplantations in China in 2019 (Hongkong, Macao and Taiwan not included)

Region	Kidney transplantation hospital	Number of patients
Tianjin	Tianjin First Central Hospital	69
Guangdong	The Second Affiliated Hospital of Guangzhou Medical University	54
Hunan	Chenzhou No.1 People's Hospital	13
Guangxi	No. 923 Hospital of the PLA Joint Logistics Support Force	11
Shandong	The Affiliated Hospital of Qingdao University	10
Beijing	Chinese PLA General Hospital	9
Hainan	The Second Affiliated Hospital of Hainan Medical University	8
Guangdong	The First Affiliated Hospital, Sun Yat-sen University	7
Shanxi	The Second People's Hospital of Shanxi Province	5
Hubei	Tongji Hospital Affiliated Tongji Medical College Huazhong University of Science and Technology	3

Recently, kidney transplantation in children (<18 years) has garnered attention. In 2019, pediatric kidney transplantations accounted for 2.9% of the total number of kidney transplantations in China (Figure 3-5).

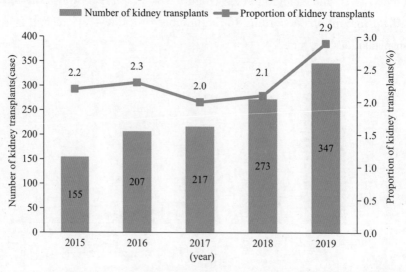

Figure 3-5　Number and proportion of kidney transplantations case during 2015–2019 in China (excluding Hong Kong, Macau, and Taiwan)

The top 5 provinces based on the number of kidney transplantations cases in 2019 were Guangdong (1,769), Hubei (1,318), Shandong (965), Zhejiang (924), and Hunan (897). The distribution of kidney transplantation cases in each province is shown below in Figure 3-6.

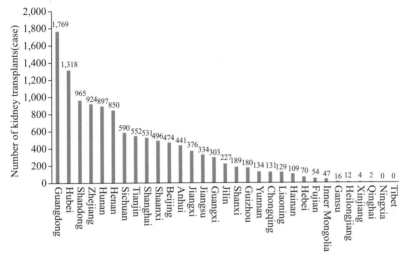

Figure 3-6　Distribution of kidney transplantation cases in each provinces of China in 2019　(excluding Hong Kong, Macau, and Taiwan)

In 2019, no less than 250 cases of kidney transplantation were performed at 14 medical institutions, which accound for 44.4% 200–249 cases were performed in 5 medical institutions, 100–199 were performed in 19 medical institutions, 50–99 were performed in 25 medical institutions, 10–49 were performed in 40 medical institutions, 1–9 were performed in 19 medical institutions, and 0 was performed in 13 medical institutions (8 of which had never performed a kidney transplantation for 3 consecutive years, from 2017 to 2019). The number and proportion of kidney transplantation cases in each range in 2019 are shown below in Talde 3-2.

In 2019, kidney transplantation demonstrated obvious regional advantages, and no less than 600 (55.5% of the total cases) cases of kidney transplantation were performed in 6 provinces of China (Figure 3-8).

Table 3-2 Number and proportion of kidney transplantation cases in each range in 2019 (Hongkong, Macao and Taiwan not included)

Range of transplantation cases	Number of medical institutions	Proportion of subjects (%)
≥250	14	44.4
200-249	5	9.1
100-199	19	21.9
50-99	25	14.7
10-49	40	9.3
1-9	19	0.6
0	13	0

Table 3-3 Distribution of kidney transplantation cases in each provime of China in 2019 (Hongkong, Macao and Taiwan not included)

Range of transplantation cases	Number of medical institutions	Proportion of subjects (%)
≥600	6	55.5
400-599	6	25.4
200-399	4	10.2
100-199	6	7.2
1-99	7	1.7
0	2	0

In 2019, the top 10 provinces based on the number of DD kidney transplantations cases in China were Guangdong (1,713), Hubei (1,264), Hunan (834), Shandong (820), Zhejiang (708), Henan (678), Tianjin (517), Shanghai (468), Shaanxi (442), and Beijing (394), which accounted for 75.4% of the total number of deceased donor kidney transplantation cases in 2019 (Figure 3-7).

In 2019, the top 5 provinces according to the number of living-related donor kidney transplantation cases were Sichuan (295), Anhui (290), Zhejiang (216), Henan (172), and Shandong(145) (Figure 3-8).

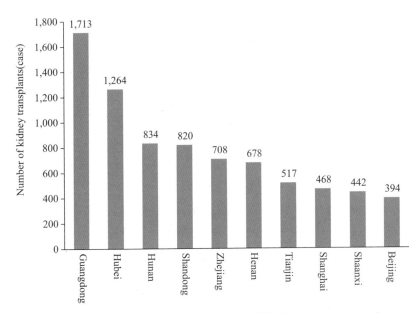

Figure 3-7　Top 10 provinces based on number of DD kidney transplantations case in 2019 (Hongkong, Macao and Taiwan not included)

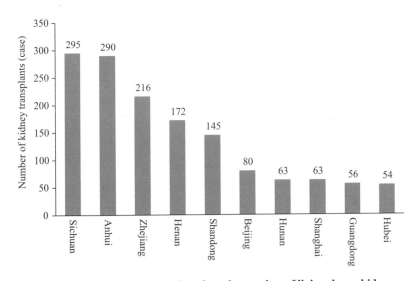

Figure 3-8　Top 10 provinces based on the number of living donor kidney transplantations cases in 2019 (Hongkong, Macao and Taiwan not included)

3.2 Data of kidney transplant recipients

The demographic analysis of the kidney transplantation cases performed in China in 2019 revealed that the recipient age was 40.1 ± 12.1 years. In addition, the analysis revealed that the value of BMI was 23.1 ± 4.3 kg/m², and the duration of pretransplant dialysis was 711 ± 876 days. In total, 70.6% of the transplant recipients were males, and the ones with AB blood type had the smallest proportion (9.0%) (Table 3-4).

Table 3-4   Basic information of kidney transplantation recipients in 2019
(Hongkong, Macao and Taiwan not included)

Variable	Mean ± SD
Recipient age (years)	40.1 ± 12.1
BMI (kg/m²)	23.1 ± 4.3
Preoperative dialysis duration (days)	771 ± 876
Recipient blood type	Proportion (%)
O	34.2
A	30.0
B	26.8
AB	9.0
Gender	Proportion (%)
Male	70.6
Female	29.4

(1) Among all recipients, 347 (2.9%), 2,062 (17.0%), 6,792 (56.0%), 2,723 (22.5%), and 200 (1.6%) were children (<18 years), 18-30 years old, 30-50 years old, 50-65 years old, and elderly (≥65 years), respectively.

(2) Pediatric donors (<18 years) accounted for 7.7%, among whom donors aged <1 year, 1-7 years, 7-12 years, and 12-18 years accounted for 15.0%, 35.5%, 20.6%, and 28.9%, respectively.

3.3　Quality and safety analysis of kidney transplantation

3.3.1　Ischemia time of donor kidney for DD kidney transplantation

An analysis of living and deceased donor kidney transplantation cases in 2019 was performed. The mean cold ischemia time for kidneys did not exceed 6 hours (Table 3-5). The cold ischemia time for 99% of living donor kidney transplants and 98.5% of deceased donor kidney transplants was ≤24 hours. The warm ischemia time for 98.1% of living donor kidney transplants and 81.3% of deceased donor kidney transplants was ≤10 minutes (Table 3-6).

Figure 3-5　Graft ischemic time in China in 2019
(Hongkong, Macao and Taiwan not included)

Variable	Living donor (mean ± standard deviation)	Deceased donor (mean ± standard deviation)
Kidney cold ischemia time (hours)	1.9 ± 1.3	5.8 ± 3.8
Kidney warm ischemia time (minutes)	3.7 ± 3.3	8.7 ± 7.4

Figure 3-6　The proportion of graft ischemia time in China in 2019
(Hongkong, Macao and Taiwan not included)

Variable	Living donor (%)	Deceased donor (%)
Kidney cold ischemia time≤24 (hours)	99.0	98.5
Kidney warm ischemia time≤10 (minutes)	98.1	81.3

3.3.2　Changes in serum creatinine values before and after kidney transplantation

In 2019, there were 12,124 cases of kidney transplantations in China. According to the requirement of CSRKT, the mean values of serum creatinine in recipients of living kidney transplantation between relatives and DD kidney transplantation at 4 follow-up time points (pre-operation, postoperative 30, 180, and 360 days) were analyzed (Figure 3-7).

Figure 3-7   Mean value of recipients' serum creatinine before and after kidney transplantationin China in 2019 (Hongkong, Macao and Taiwan not included)

Time point	Living donor (μmol/L)	Deceased donor (μmol/L)
Before surgery	986.7	914.2
30 days after surgery	119.4	150.0
180 days after surgery	115.0	123.5
360 days after surgery	119.5	115.6

3.2.3   Overview of adverse events after kidney transplantation

Significant adverse events after kidney transplantation usually include delayed function of allograft, acute rejection, death of recipient, and renal allograft loss. According to the retrospective analysis of cases in 2019, the incidence of significant adverse events is presented in Table 3-8 and 3-9. The 30-day postoperative mortality rate was 0.4%. Not major complication wasshowed in the living organ donors within postoperative 30 days.

Table 3-8   Incidence of adverse events within postoperative in China in 2019 (Hongkong, Macao and Taiwan not included)

Adverse event	Living donor kidney transplantation (%)	DD kidney transplantation (%)
Delayed ograft function	1.3	8.7
Acute rejection	3.2	3.1
Infection	3.7	5.9
Recipient death	0.5	1.2
All-cause graft loss	1.2	4.3

Table 3-9   Incidences of adverse events after combined pancreas-kidney transplantation in China in 2019 (Hongkong, Macao and Taiwan not included)

Adverse event	Overall incidence (%)
Delayed ograft function	2.7
Acute rejection	10.1
Infection	20.1
Recipient death	4.0
All-cause graft loss	5.4

3.3.4 Survival analysis of kidney transplant recipient and graft

A survival analysis was performed for recipients and grafts (hereinafter patient/kidney) for 52,005 kidney transplantation cases in China from 2015 to 2019.

(1) 1-year survival probability after transplantation: the 1-year survival probability of recipient/allograft was 97.8% / 95.7%, whereas the survival probabilities of recipient and graft were 94.4% / 98.8%, respectively (Table 3-10).

(2) 3-year survival probability after transplantation: the 3-year survival probability of recipient/allograft after DD kidney transplantation was 96.9% / 93.3%, whereas the 3-year survival probability of recipient/allograft after living relative donor kidney transplantation was 98.9% / 97.0% (Table 3-10).

Table 3-10   Survival probabilities of kidney transplant recipient and graft after kidney transplantation in China (Hongkong, Macao and Taiwan not included)

Donortype	1-year		3-year	
	Recipient (%)	Allograft (%)	Recipient (%)	Allograft (%)
DD	97.8	95.7	96.9	93.3
Living donor	99.4	98.8	98.9	97.0

3.4 Summary and prospects

1. Deceased donor kidney transplantation is the main type of transplantation at present

Since 2015, organ donation from deceased donors has been greatly encouraged in China. In 2019, the proportion of deceased donor kidney transplantations was 85.7%; furthermore, Guangdong, Hubei, Shandong, Zhejiang, and Hunan were the top provinces according to the number of kidney transplantation cases, showing significant regional dominance. Recently, Guangdong, Henan, and Shanghai have performed the most pediatric kidney transplants. In addition, pediatric kidney donors accounted for 7.7% of all kidney donors in China in 2019.

The region allocation principle for organs and the establishment of green channels for organ transport have shortened the cold ischemia time for deceased donor kidney transplantation. The 1-year and 3-year graft survival rates for living and deceased donor kidney transplants are satisfactory. In 2019, 66.5% of 224 kidney-related combined multi-organ transplantations were combined pancreas-kidney transplantations, which were mostly performed in Tianjin, Guangdong, Hunan, Guangxi, and Shandong.

3.4.2　Quality control and improvement project of kidney transplantation has been conducted

The central principles for quality control are to set up a system matching the developmental characteristics of kidney transplantation in China, achieve industrial leadership, strengthen the management of human organ transplantation medical quality, achieve continuous improvement in the national medical quality of kidney transplantation and service levels, and decrease medical gaps in various transplantation centers. Therefore, a series of quality control criteria and technical specifications were developed. In addition, these technical formulations were used to establish a kidney transplantation quality improvement process, and prospective studies were conducted, thereby achieving a virtuous cycle of medical quality assessment (control) to medical quality improvement, which continuously drives the development of the kidney transplantation industry in China.

3.4.3　Attention has been paid to the hot issues in kidney transplantation and breakthroughs have beenmade

The shortage of donors and allograft rejection in organ transplantation will still be the key constrained factors of the development of kidney transplantation for a long period to come. Over the years, domestic scholars have been committed to linking the research results in immunology, stem cell, and genetic engineering with the organ transplantation, and carrying out basic and clinical research works, in order to provide the theoretical and practical basis for improving the medical quality of kidney transplantation. There have been several breakthroughs, such as donor-specific antibody, antibody-mediated rejection, clinical immune tolerance, organ function maintenance for potential organ donor, preservation and full utilization of donated organ, and transplantation-related virus infections, in research hotspots.

3.4.4   Letting the international transplantation community hear the "Voice of China"

CSRKT is the precious wealth of China in organ transplantation. In order to make the CSRKT more scientific and modernized, the Kidney Transplantation Quality Control Center has also mined the data of the CSRKT and performed a large sample, real-world study of the clinical outcomes of Chinese kidney transplant recipients. The research report, which was presented at European Congress of the Transplantation Society, and published in the international journal, *Transplant International* revealed the characteristics, achievements, shortcomings, and prospects of kidney transplantation in the Mainland China. It has not only raised the voice of China in transplantation in the big data atmosphere, but also strengthened the academic exchanges in the international transplantation, thereby providing a scientific foundation for the sustainable and healthy development of kidney transplantation in China. In addition, the journal published a commentary highlighting that we "should praise the outstanding achievements of transplantation work in China". In addition, the quality control center submitted manuscripts to the *World Medical Journal and Chinese Medical Journal*, which factually describe the experience of the growth of the Chinese organ transplantation system under exploratory specifications, enabling the international medical community to hear the "Voice of China". The facts of China's organ transplantation development are used to refute fallacies by some organizations with ulterior motives to politicize transplantation and show that China's organ transplantation workers will continuously improve to develop China's organ transplantation industry complying with the ethics and standards of the World Health Organization.

Chapter 4　Heart Transplantation in China

This chapter is mainly based on the data of China Heart Transplant Registry (CHTR).

CHTR is established under the supervision of the National Health Commission as an official heart transplant registry system, and it requires the medical institutions with heart transplantation qualifications to submit heart transplantation data.

CHTR included characteristics of recipient, donor and transplant, immunosuppressants, in-hospital and long-term outcomes.

CHTR releases regular reports regarding the national, regional, and center-specific heart transplantation volumes, results of data audit, and patient outcomes via comprehensive analysis of collected data. Based on those analyses and reports, CHTR summaries results and experience on heart donor acquisition and preservation, donor-recipients matching and clinical transplantation management. Furthermore, CHTR provides vital information for the constitution of relative regulations, laws and guidelines for the relative national administrative.

4.1　Distribution of medical institutions for heart transplantation

By December 31, 2019, a total of 57 medical institutions were qualified for heart transplantation in China, which was an increase of 11 medical institutions compared with that in 2018. Provinces with the most number of such medical institutions with heart transplantation qualifications were Guangdong (6), Zhejiang (6), Beijing (5), and Hubei (5) (Figure 4-1).

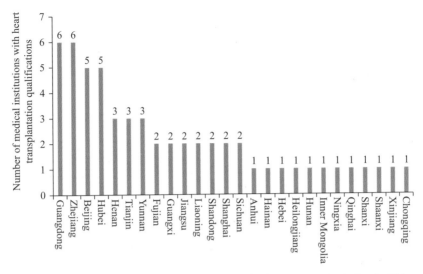

Figure 4-1　Distribution of medical institutions for heart transplantation in China in 2019 (Hongkong, Macao and Taiwan not included)

As revealed by CHTR 2,262 heart transplantation cases were performed in China during 2015–2019 (Figure 4-2). In 2019, 679 cases heart transplantation were complete in 38 medical institutions qualified for heart transplantation. This was a 38.6% increase in the number of transplantation cases compared with that in 2018. Among these cases, 59 were pediatric (<18 years) heart transplantations and 8 were combined heart-lung transplantations. Figure 4-3 shows the distribution of heart transplantation cases in the provinces. Figure 4-4 shows the top 10 medical institutions according to the number of heart transplantations in China (HongKong, Macao, and Taiwan not included) in 2019.

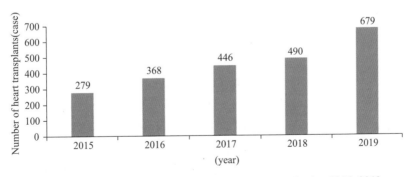

Figure 4-2　Number of heart transplantation cases during 2015–2019 (Hongkong, Macao and Taiwan not included)

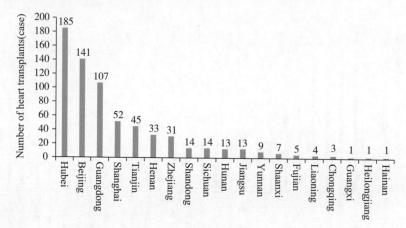

Figure 4-3 **Distribution of heart transplantation cases in each provinces of China in 2019 (Hongkong, Macao and Taiwan not included)**

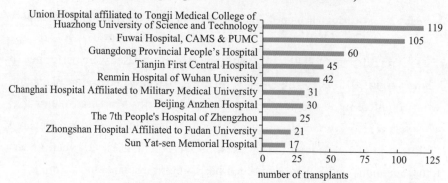

Figure 4-4 **Top 10 medical institutions by the number of transplantation cases in 2019 (Hongkong, Macao and Taiwan not included)**

4.2 Demographic characteristics of heart transplantation recipients

In 2019, the median age of heart transplantation recipients was 50 years. Male recipients accounted for 74.7% of all heart transplantation recipients in China, and the median BMI of these recipients was 22.3 kg/m^2. The proportions of heart transplantation recipients with O, A, B, and AB blood types were 30.8%, 30.5%, 28.3%, and 10.4%, respectively. The median age of pediatric heart transplantation recipients was 11 years, and males accounted for

49.1% of all pediatric heart transplantation recipients in China (Table 4-1). The main causes for heart transplantation were nonischemic cardiomyopathy and coronary heart disease, which accounted for 71.0% and 13.7%, respectively, followed by congenital heart disease (4.3%), valvular heart disease (5.7%), and other causes (5.3%). The main causes of heart transplantation in pediatric recipients were nonischemic cardiomyopathy (76.4%) and congenital heart disease (14.6%).

Table 4-1   Demographic characteristics of heart transplantation recipients in China in 2019 (Hongkong, Macao and Taiwan not included)

Variable	All transplantation recipients	Pediatric transplantation recipients
Median age, IQR (years)	50.0 (35.0-57.0)	11.0 (7.0-14.0)
Ratio of sex/males (%)	74.7	49.1
Median weight, IQR (kg)	62.5 (52.0-71.0)	35.0 (23.0-46.0)
Median height, IQR (cm)	168.0 (162.0-173.0)	150.0 (122.0-164.0)
Median BMI, IQR (kg/m^2)	22.2 (19.4-24.5)	16.1 (13.9-18.9)
Heart transplantation etiology (%)		
Nonischemic cardiomyopathy	71.0	76.4
Coronary heart disease	13.7	0.0
Congenital heart disease	4.3	14.6
Valvular heart disease	5.7	3.6
Other diseases	5.3	5.4

Note: IQR, interquartile range

4.3   Quality and safety analysis of heart transplantation

4.3.1   Ischemia time of heart donor

Figure 4-5 shows the distribution of ischemia times for heart transplantation in 2019. In 2019, the median ischemia time for heart transplantation in China was 4.0 hours. The proportion of heart transplantation recipients with an ischemia time of more than 6 hours was 15.6%, which was 22.1% lower than that in 2015–2018.

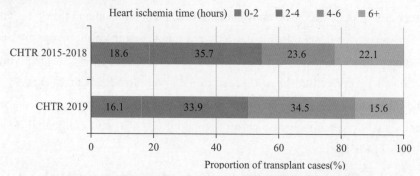

Figure 4-5   Heart ischemia time of heart transplantation in China
in 2019 (Hongkong, Macao and Taiwan not included)

4.3.2   Postoperative intra–hospital survival

In 2019, the intra-hospital survival rate of heart transplantation recipients in China was 93.2%. Among these patients, the intra-hospital survival rates of recipients who underwent heart transplantation for cardiomyopathy and coronary heart disease were 94.3% and 91.4%, respectively. The incidence of postoperative infection among heart transplant recipients was 22.0%. Other major postoperative complications include cardiac arrest (3.5%), second open-chest surgery (5.3%), tracheotomy (4.7%), and second intubation (6.0%). Among the causes of intra-hospital death among heart transplantation recipients, multi-organ failure and graft failure accounted for more than 50% of early deaths (Table 4-2).

Table 4-2   Postoperative intra-hospital survival rate of recipients after heart
transplantation of China in 2019

Variable	Rate/composition (%)
Intra-hospital survival	93.2
Postoperative complication	
Postoperative infection	22.0
Cardiac arrest	3.5
Second open-chest surgery	5.3
Tracheotomy	4.7
Second intubation	6.0

Cause of intra-hospital death	
Multi-organ failure	39.6
Graft failure	12.5
Infection	16.7
Others	31.3

4.3.3　Survival analysis

During 2015–2019, the postoperative 1-year and 3-year survival rates among recipients after heart transplantation were 85.2% and 80.0%, respectively. Among these patients, the postoperative 1-year and 3-year survival rates of adult patients after heart transplantation were 84.7% and 79.4%, respectively. The postoperative 1-year and 3-year survival rates after heart transplantation for pediatric patients were 92.6% and 90.6%, respectively (Table 4-3).

Table 4-3　Ostoperative survival rate after heart transplantation during 2015–2019 in China

	Postoperative 1-year survival rate (%)	Postoperative 3-year survival rate (%)
Total	85.2	80.0
Adults	84.7	79.4
Children	92.6	90.6

4.4　Summary and prospects

In 2019, the number of heart transplantation cases increased rapidly as evidenced by an increase of 38.6% compared with that in 2018. In 2019, 11 medical institutions that possessed heart transplantation qualifications were added, showing that the regional accessibility of heart transplantation in China is gradually increasing. In 2019, heart transplantation centers in 3 hospitals, including the Union Hospital affiliated to the Tongji Medical College of Huazhong University of Science and Technology, Fuwai Hospital of the

Chinese Academy of Medical Sciences, and Guangdong Provincial People's Hospital performed 60 or more heart transplantations. This shows that 3 heart transplantation centers in China are considered international major heart transplantation centers.

As the number of heart transplantation cases rapidly increased, the intra-hospital survival rate and long-term survival rate of heart transplantation recipients in China steadily increased in 2019. Regarding heart transplant ischemia time, efficient operation of the human organ allocation and sharing computer system along with continuous efforts by various transplantation medical teams in China has drastically decreased the proportion of patients with a heart ischemia time of more than six hours. The aforementioned results show that China has accumulated successful experiences in the selection and maintenance of heart transplants, perioperative management of recipients, and postoperative long-term management.

In 2019, the committee of national heart transplantation quality control center revised and published the 2019 Technical Specifications for Heart Transplantation Diagnosis and Treatment. These specifications cover preoperative assessment and preparation of heart transplantation recipients; heart transplantation operation procedures; immunosuppressant treatment; rejection reaction diagnosis and treatment; diagnosis and treatment of postoperative complications; and postoperative follow-up. Simultaneously, academic seminars and technical qualification training were used to explain technical specifications to further improve the homogenization of heart transplantation-related techniques in China.

In the future, the national heart transplantation quality control center will further improve the registration system for heart transplantation in China and establish an international collaboration and exchange system. Expert committee meetings will be conducted to develop heart transplantation-related quality control systems and technical specifications, strengthen the technical training of heart transplantation-related techniques, support hospitals which were week in technology and management, and gradually reduce interregional differences.

Chapter 5 Lung Transplantation in China

The data analyzed in this chapter are of those patients registered by each lung transplantation center in China Lung Transplantation Registry (CLuTR) from January 1, 2015 to December 31, 2018. As the unique scientific registry system of lung transplant data in China, CLuTR has comprehensively and timely collected the preoperative information of recipients, donor information, transplantation information of recipients, postoperative information, and follow-up information. By dynamic and scientific analysis of the lung transplantation in Mainland China, CLuTR provides a basis for national regulatory authorities to formulate the relevant transplantation policies and regulations.

5.1 Distribution of medical institutions for lung transplantation

During 2015–2019, 43 medical institutions in China have obtained qualifications for lung transplantation. These institutions covered 21 provinces in China and were mainly concentrated in eastern and northern China. However, Hebei, Shanxi, Jilin, Jiangxi, Chongqing, Guizhou, Tibet, Gansu, Qinghai, and Ningxia had no medical institutions that obtained lung transplantation qualifications (Figure 5-1).

From January 1, 2015 to December 31, 2019, 1,513 cases of lung transplantation were reported by CLuTR, including 118 cases in 2015, 204 cases in 2016, 299 cases in 2017, 403 cases in 2018, 489 cases in 2019 (Figure 5-2), showing an upward trend year by year.

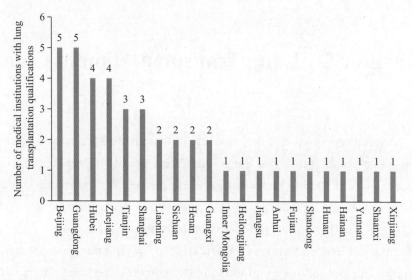

Figure 5-1   Distribution of medical institutions qualified for lung transplantation in each province of China in 2019 (Hongkong, Macao and Taiwan not included)

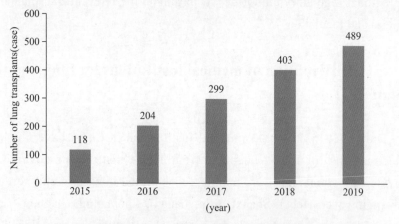

Figure 5-2   Number of lung transplantation during 2015–2018 in China (Hongkong, Macao and Taiwan not included)

In 2019, lung transplantation was performed in 23 centers. The top 3 centers by the number of operations were Wuxi People's Hospital (30.5%), China-Japan Friendship Hospital (20.0%), and the First Affiliated Hospital of Guangzhou Medical University (16.1%) (Figure 5-3).

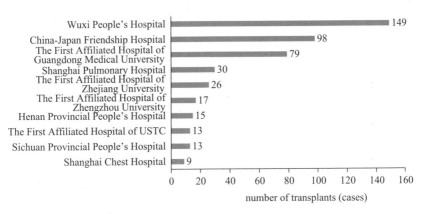

Figure 5-3   Top 10 medical institutions by the number of lung transplantation cases in 2019 in China (Hongkong, Macao and Taiwan not included)

5.2 Demographic characteristics of lung transplantation recipients

In 2019, the median (interquartile range (IQR)) ischemia times for single and double lung transplantations in China were 6.0 (4.0-7.0) and 8.0 (6.2-9.3) hours, respectively. The proportions of patients with cold ischemia time of <2 h, 2-4 h, 4-6 h, 6-8 h, and ≥8 h among all single lung transplantation patients were 4.3%, 27.5%, 24.9%, 37.7%, and 5.6%, respectively. Furthermore, the proportion of patients with cold ischemia time of <2h, 2-4h, 4-6h, 6-8h, and ≥8h among all double lung transplantation patients were 2.2%, 6.6%, 15.8%, 30.1%, and 45.3%, respectively (Figure 5-4).

In 2019, males accounted for 82.2% of all lung transplantation recipients in China. The mean age was 54.9 ± 12.8 years, and 49.0% of all lung transplantation recipients were aged 60 years and above. The mean BMI of these recipients was 20.3 ± 3.9 kg/m². The proportions of recipients with O, A, B, and AB blood types were 29.6%, 32.3%, 30.2%, and 7.9%, respectively. Before transplantation, 29.6% of all recipients were treated with steroids and 9.4% were admitted to the intensive care unit (ICU). The proportions of recipients with complete limitation to activities of daily living (NYHA IV) and those with severe disease requiring inpatient treatment were 15.6% and 12.5%, respectively (Table 5-1).

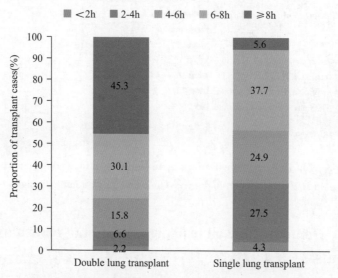

Figure 5-4   Cold ischemia times of single and double lung transplantation patients in China in 2019 (Hongkong, Macao and Taiwan not included)

Table 5-1   Demographic characteristics of lung transplantation recipients in China in 2019 (Hongkong, Macao and Taiwan not included)

Variable	Proportion (%)
Sex	
Male	82.2
Female	17.8
Age (years)	
<18	1.8
18-35	10.0
36-49	15.7
50-59	23.5
60-64	27.7
≥65	21.3

Variable	Proportion (%)
BMI (kg/m^2)	
<18.5	33.5
18.6-23.9	46.0
≥24.0	20.5
Blood type	
O	29.6
A	32.3
B	30.2
AB	7.9
Steroid treatment history	
Present	29.6
Absent	70.4
Pre-transplantation hospitalization status	
ICU	9.4
Normal hospitalization	75.1
Not hospitalized	15.5
Pre-transplantation cardiac function status	
No limitation in activities of daily living (NYHA I/II)	1.4
Partial limitation in activities of daily living (NYHA III)	70.5
Complete limitation in activities of daily living (NYHA IV)	15.6
Severe disease requiring inpatient treatment	12.5

In 2019, the causes for lung transplantation in China were mainly idiopathic interstitial pneumonia, chronic obstructive pulmonary disease, secondary interstitial pneumonia, and pneumoconiosis, which accounted for 37.0%, 20.9%, 11.0%, 10.2% of all cases, respectively. In addition, bronchiectasis, pulmonary hypertension, obliterative bronchiolitis, lung transplant failure, and lymphangioleiomyomatosis accounted for 7.8%, 3.1%, 2.2%, 1.2%, and 1.0% of all cases, respectively (Figure 5-5).

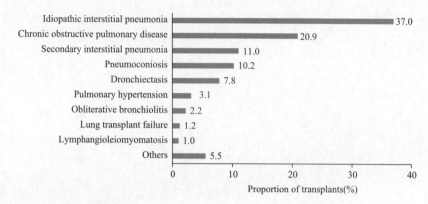

**Figure 5-5   Distribution of primary causes of lung transplantation in China
in 2019 (Hongkong, Macao and Taiwan not included)**

5.3   Quality and safety analysis of lung transplantation

5.3.1   Surgery procedure

In 2019, single and double lung transplantations accounted for 45.0% and 55.0% of all lung transplantations in China, respectively. Emergency lung transplantation accounted for 14.0%, and the proportion of patients who required intraoperative extracorporeal membrane oxygenation (Extracorporeal Membrane Oxygenation, ECMO) was 60.2%.

5.3.2   Intraoperative blood transfusion

The proportion of patients with median intraoperative blood transfusion volume (IQR) of 1,065.0 mL (600.0-1,790.0 mL), < 500 mL, 500-999 mL, 1,000-1,499 mL, 1,500-1,999 mL, and ≥2,000 mL was 18.6%, 23.7%, 21.1%, 15.1%, and 21.5%, respectively.

5.3.3   Early postoperative complications (< 30 days)

Early postoperative complications mainly include infection (65.2%), renal insufficiency (30.9%), primary lung graft failure (18.3%), diabetes (15.9%), acute rejection (8.4%), and tracheal anastomotic lesion (6.4%) (Figure 5-6).

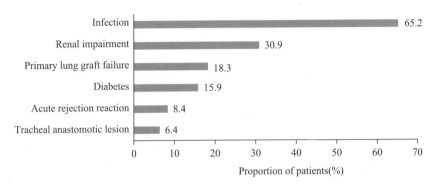

Figure 5-6   Perioperative complications among lung transplantation recipients in China in 2019 (Hongkong, Macao and Taiwan not included)

5.3.4   Discharge status

In 2019, the median (IQR) length of hospitalization among lung transplantation recipients in China was 30.0 days (19.0-49.0 days), and the predischarge survival rate was 75.8%. The main causes of perioperative death in recipients were shock or respiratory failure caused by infection (27.7%), multi-organ failure (27.7%), primary lung graft failure (13.8%), and sudden cardiac death (10.8%) (Figure 5-7).

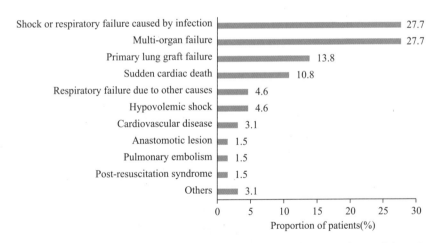

Figure 5-7   Causes of perioperative death among lung transplantation recipients in China in 2019 (Hongkong, Macao and Taiwan not included)

5.3.5 Postoperative survival

In China, the postoperative (<30 days), 3-month, 6-month, 1-year, and 3-year survival rates of patients receiving double-lung transplantation were 78.8%, 69.3%, 65.3%, 63.5%, and 56.1%, respectively, for double lung transplantation recipients and 84.2%, 77.7%, 73.5%, 68.7%, and 52.3%, respectively, for single lung transplantation recipients. The short-term survival rate for single lung transplantation recipients was better than that for double lung transplantation recipients (Table 5-2).

Table 5-2　Survival rate of recipients after lung transplantation surgery in China (Hongkong, Macao and Taiwan not included)

	Perioperative period (<30 days)	3-months	6-months	1-year	3-years
Double lung (%)	78.8	69.3	65.3	63.5	56.1
Single lung (%)	84.2	77.7	73.5	68.7	52.3

5.4　Summary and prospects

Recently, the national lung transplantation quality control center has continuously upgraded the clinical diagnosis and treatment system for lung transplantation and promoted standardized lung transplantation techniques. The number of lung transplantation patients in China increased rapidly in 2019 compared with that in 2018, and the increasing trend in the number of lung transplants was maintained. In 2019, major improvements and breakthroughs were achieved in pediatric lung transplantation, but the incidence of emergency lung transplantation, postoperative infection, primary graft failure, sudden cardiac death, renal impairment, and postoperative complication is still high.

5.4.1　The first international lung transplantation forum in China was successfully held and promoted the early entry of lung transplantation in China to the international stage

On November 2, 2019, the first international lung transplantation forum in China was successfully held in Wuxi. The forum attracted thoracic cardiovascular surgery experts and professors from the Cleveland Clinic in USA, Faculty of Medicine of the University of Milan in Italy, Faculty of Medicine of the University of Tokyo in Japan, and Asan Medical Center and University of Ulsan College of Medicine in South Korea along with cardiothoracic surgery experts from Queen Mary Hospital in Hong Kong and Linkou Chang Gung Memorial Hospital in Taiwan. The forum discussed topics on internal medicine and surgical techniques, anesthesia, nursing, basic research experiences, and new developments in lung transplantation, and diverse academic activities with rich content such as case exchange and discussion were performed. This forum provided opportunities for a high-level exchange of knowledge and skills between Chinese and international lung transplantation experts and helped drive the continuous development of the transplantation industry in China. In the future, China's lung transplantation industry will be further connected internationally and be better integrated into the large international transplantation family to make major contributions in medical science.

5.4.2   Continuous improvement in pediatric lung transplantation techniques

Presently, pediatric lung transplantation remains a bottleneck in lung transplantation in China. From 2015 to 2018, 8 pediatric lung transplantations in children aged below 18 years were performed in the entire country. The perioperative survival rate was still poor. However, 9 pediatric lung transplantations were completed in 2019, which set records for the youngest pediatric lung transplantation in China and the most number of pediatric lung transplantations in a year. Presently, the overall conditions of the pediatric recipients remain good. Due to large differences in physical function, growth and development, and immune rejection between children and adults, many technical difficulties remain in the clinical management of pediatric lung transplantation needing to be overcome.

5.4.3 Implementation of pre-lung transplantation assessment system and reducing emergency lung transplantation

The preoperative cardiac function and proportion of ICU admissions among lung transplantation recipients were lower, but the proportion of emergency lung transplantation cases was higher in 2019 than those in 2015–2018. Due to their severe conditions and time constraints, acute lung transplantation patients have higher risks of postoperative rejection and primary graft failure, and the postoperative perioperative survival rate and short-term and long-term survival rates among these patients are lower. Therefore, a pre-lung transplantation assessment system should be further promoted to strictly manage transplantation contraindications and indications among recipients.

5.3.4 Strengthening postoperative complication monitoring and control

In 2019, the incidence of infections after lung transplantation was comparable to those of the preceding years. However, the incidence of primary graft failure, sudden cardiac death, and renal insufficiency significantly increased. A whole process and multi-aspect infection control system should be established to achieve good infection prevention and control through preoperative assessment, donor quality maintenance, surgical procedure, and postoperative management. Regarding the prevention and control of primary graft failure, donor quality should be maintained, and cardiopulmonary bypass should be considered or ECMO duration can be extended for recipients with poor physical conditions. Regarding the prevention of sudden cardiac death, preoperative assessment of cardiac function should be emphasized, and postoperative dynamic monitoring of cardiac function should be performed. Aggressive treatment should be provided for recipients with abnormal cardiac function. Regarding the prevention of renal insufficiency, attention should be paid to the monitoring of drug concentration and renal function markers, particularly drug-drug interactions, to reduce kidney burden as much as possible.

Even though lung transplantation has experienced rapid development in China recently, the survival rates in China are significantly different compared with those reported by the International Society for Heart and Lung Transplantation. The main reason for this phenomenon is that lung transplantation recipients in China are older and in more critical conditions, surgery difficulty is higher, there are more patients with pulmonary fibrosis, ventilator usage duration for deceased donor lungs is longer, and cold ischemia time is longer than those internationally. In the future, the lung transplantation quality control center will further revise the clinical application quality control markers for lung transplantation techniques, improve lung transplantation standard procedures and technical specifications, continuously establish multidisciplinary lung transplantation teams, construct a complete lung transplantation database, mine data resources, and continuously upgrade the quality of lung transplantation.